MEDICINAL MUSHROOMS

MEDICINAL MUSHROOMS

Ancient Remedies for Modern Ailments

Georges M. Halpern, M.D.
and Andrew H. Miller

M. EVANS AND COMPANY, INC.
New York

DISCLAIMER

This book contains reports of studies and anecdotal accounts concerning medicinal mushrooms. The information reported herein is derived from sources believed to be reliable. However, the authors do not warrant the adequacy or accuracy of these studies or accounts. The authors are not providing medical advice. Anyone with any of the medical conditions discussed herein should seek medical treatment and not attempt to self-cure with the use of medicinal mushrooms alone. Do not attempt to self-medicate for potentially serious medical conditions without medical supervision.

Medicinal mushrooms, like other herbal supplements, are not regulated by the US Food and Drug Administration (FDA). No statement contained herein has been evaluated by the FDA. The products mentioned herein are not intended to diagnose, treat, cure, or prevent any disease. All herbal supplements have both benefits and risks. Information about long-term side effects and interactions is incomplete. The reader should not assume that because an adverse reaction or interaction is not mentioned in this book, the use of medicinal mushrooms is always safe. If you suspect you could be experiencing an adverse reaction from an herb or a combination of herbs and drugs, you should immediately consult with a health professional.

The authors, several mycologists, and several companies mentioned in the book transact business with each other, and have financial interests in some of the entities mentioned herein. The authors have accepted no promotional money in exchange for the endorsement of any product herein.

M. Evans and Company, Inc.
216 East 49th Street
New York, New York 10017

Library of Congress Cataloging-in-Publication Data

Miller, Andrew
    Medicinal mushroom : ancient remedies for modern ailments /
    [Andrew Miller, Gorges Halpern]
       p.   cm.
    Includes bibliographical references and index.
    ISBN 0-87131981-0 (alk. paper)
    1. Mushrooms—Therapeutic use. I. Halpern, Gerges M. II. Title.
RM666.M87 M54 2002
615'.3296—cd21   2002067737

Watercolors by Marie Heerkens
Book design and typesetting by Terry Bain
Printed in the United States of America
9   8   7   6   5   4   3   2   1

Table of Contents

Acknowledgments

My father was a mycologist by necessity: He had to find food when he was close to starvation in Eastern Galicia during his childhood, and in Siberia during the family exile of 1916. He taught me about the *cèpes*, chanterelles, and *trompettes-de-la-mort* when we were hiding from the French police and the Gestapo in the Ardèche in 1941, and around Aigue-belette in 1942. It was then I discovered the shapes, the colors, the taste, and the magic of marvelous and accessible foods. During the short breaks outside the refugee camps in Switzerland, I found myself hoping for rain during the late summer or early fall, and would crawl back to the hidden, secret circles where these delicious mushrooms would sprout, sending their odoriferous messages to be captured only by the initiated.

My next experience with mushrooms was my initiation to the medicinal properties of *Psylocybes* during my residency as a shrink; we did not jump, fly, or get sick. We just discovered a new world, shared with the *curanderas* and our schizophrenic patients. But Tomio Toda, the immunologist and Noh Master, was promoting *Lentinula edodes*, the shiitake mushroom, as an immunostimulant against "our" *Corynebacterium parvum*. Soon, Lentinan, the stimulant made from shiitake, would be a major drug in Japan.

My attraction to mushrooms was justified, and my quest would take me to the Pacific Rim: Asia and California. Here we are, and I must thank Norman Goldfind, my agent, for helping us with this volume; George de Kay, the publisher, is confident and will help for the success of this book. Peter Weverka provided his time, research, skills, humor, patience, and typing skills: he *made* this book. I cannot forget my wife and daughters, not because they escaped too often the fate of Sacha Guitry's own as described in the first pages of his *Roman d'un Tricheur*, but simply because they still love me despite the long physical and mental absences.

Georges Halpern, M.D., Ph.D.
Portola Valley, California
January, 2002

On a brilliant, sunny Los Angeles morning in the summer of 1987, while on a business trip searching for new products and suppliers for my Chinese herbal products company, I found myself in a small herb shop in Venice Beach. Surrounded by large glass vessels of exotic-looking botanicals and shelves full of packaged tonics treasured for centuries as agents of radiant health, I found myself mesmerized by the oratory of the owner, who went on at length about the life-transforming qualities of a large red mushroom called reishi, known as the mushroom of immortality by the ancient Taoists and spiritual adepts of the Orient.

A spore was planted in my mind that day; it took root and germinated into a fifteen-year journey exploring the benefits, research, cultivation technologies, and art of medicinal mushrooms. It has been a fascinating time for me, and I have met many dedicated and wonderful people along the way. I would like to acknowledge their support and contributions here.

Special thanks goes to Dr. E. J. Wilson, Jr., who has been a loyal, kind, and great business partner for almost two decades and who has pioneered brilliant and novel technologies for preparing medicinal mushrooms for increased bioavailability, potency, and benefit for the consumer.

Thanks to Dr. Randy Dorian of Hanuman Medical and Dr. Moshe Shifrine for their support and collaboration on working toward the advancement of liquid culture medicinal mushroom cultivation. Their art will benefit many, many people as the value of medicinal mushrooms becomes more and more recognized. Thanks to Jordan Rubin for his wealth of knowledge, good cheer, and positive attitude. Of course, Dr. Georges Halpern, friend and colleague, who encouraged me to collaborate with him on this book and to share my experiences and knowledge to help further the cause. Thank you to Peter Weverka, friend and fellow carpooler, who was the glue that cemented the ideas and text of this book. Thanks to all those who helped along the way, and especially to Thomas Hickey, whose sudden passing has taken us by surprise. As president of Tea Garden Products, Inc., he brought a degree of professionalism and ethical conduct to our industry that was admired by many. I will miss his insightful comments and long conversations about medicinal mushrooms and Chinese herbs. Last but not least, to my wife, Martine, and daughters, Louise and Pauline, who have always been my strongest inspiration to be and do the best I can.

Andrew H. Miller
San Francisco, California
June, 2002

Introduction

Medicinal Mushrooms: Ancient Remedies for Modern Ailments is dedicated to bringing information about the healing powers of medicinal mushrooms to Western readers. Some of the mushrooms described in this book have been used as medicines for two thousand years or more. Others were discovered in recent decades. All have medicinal properties that can improve your health and well-being.

For the general reader, this book presents the fascinating history of eight medicinal mushrooms: reishi, *Cordyceps sinensis, Agaricus blazei,* maitake, *Phellinus linteus, Trametes versicolor, Hericium erinaceus,* and shiitake. This book explains how ancient people used these medicinal mushrooms and the promise they bring for healing and preventing illness in the modern world. For the general reader, we have strived to put a human face on a subject that is too often dry and clinical. In these pages you will find behind-the-scenes stories about the mycologists and scientists who are bringing medicinal mushrooms into the world at large. Where we describe the action of medicinal mushrooms on the body, we have done our best to do so in terms that the layman can understand.

For the reader who is already a student of medicinal mushrooms, this book presents the latest scientific and clinical research. It describes the most up-to-date experiments and conjectures how different medicinal mushrooms may be used to treat and prevent illness.

Our Approach to This Subject

Many claims are made for medicinal mushrooms. Sometimes out of sheer enthusiasm and sometimes for commercial motives, authors make exaggerated claims. A few of these claims border on the outlandish. For example, the label on a medicinal mushroom product we have (it comes from China) claims the following: "Effective on cancer, AIDS, hepatitis, headaches, colds, and impotence." Claims like these raise false hopes. Worse, they give people cause to be cynical about medicinal mushrooms and herbal remedies in general.

For this book, we chose to exercise skepticism. We were careful to examine sources of information to make sure that they were reliable. Except for historical purposes, we have endeavored to cite only studies and experiments that were undertaken in the past five or six years. We want to present the most current information about medicinal mushrooms. In the back of this book, you will find references listed under chapter headings, in case you are interested in looking further into a study we cite.

No medicinal mushroom is a cure-all. No mushroom can sweep away disease in everyone who takes it. No mushroom can make the body unassailable to disease. What mushrooms can do is bolster the immune system. They can give a powerful boost to the functions of the body that are already in place for preventing and fighting disease. In this book, we take the balanced view. We are firm believers in the medicinal properties of mushrooms, but we believe that only a balanced view can sway the skeptics, convince the doubters, and promote medicinal mushrooms as a means of healing the body and preventing disease.

What You Will Find in This Book

Chapter One looks at mushrooms in Eastern and Western culture, how they have been revered and reviled, and the role of fungi in nature. Fungi live on the most trying layer of the ecosystem, where they are constantly under attack from disease-causing pathogens. Some scientists believe that the ability of fungi to battle pathogens is what makes them beneficial to the human immune system. Because the use of mushrooms in traditional Chinese medicine is mentioned throughout this book, Chapter One also takes a quick look at traditional Chinese medicine.

As you will discover, mushrooms can make you healthy in many different ways, but they do so chiefly by awakening the immune system and making it more alert. Throughout this book, we refer to different parts of the immune system—cytokines, T cells, the lymphatic system, macrophages, and so on. Unless you are a student of biology or medicinal mushrooms, the terminology of the immune system is sure to baffle or confuse you. For that reason, Chapter Two explains the general workings of the immune system and how medicinal mushrooms awaken and restore it. We felt it was necessary to explain the immune system in some depth. Without knowing how the immune system works, it is hard to grasp how medicinal mushrooms improve your health.

Chapter Three is the first of eight chapters about medicinal mushrooms. Each chapter presents the latest scientific studies conducted on a specific medicinal mushroom. Each chapter describes a mushroom's character, the history of its use as a medicine, its healing properties, and its folklore. In the "Producer's List" near the end of this book, you will find the names, addresses, and phone numbers of companies that sell the medicinal mushroom you have been reading about.

Chapter Three is about reishi, the "mushroom of immortality," its use by ancient Taoist priests, and its antitumor and antioxidant effects. Chapter Four describes *Cordyceps sinensis,* the anti-aging and stamina-building mushroom that generated so many headlines in 1993 when the coach of the Chinese women's track team credited it for helping his runners break three world records in a single week. Chapter Five concerns *Agaricus blazei,* the unusual mushroom from Brazil that many believe has the strongest antitumor activity.

In Chapter Six, you will read about maitake, a delicious culinary mushroom that lowers cholesterol and helps against diabetes, among other things. Chapter Seven looks at *Phellinus linteus,* a mushroom that has long been cherished in Korea as an aid against stomach ailments and arthritis. Chapter Eight examines *Trametes versicolor,* the mushroom from which Krestin, one of the world's foremost anticancer drugs, is derived. Chapter Nine delves into *Hericium erinaceus,* a mushroom that may hold promise as a cure for Alzheimer's disease. The last of the mushroom chapters, Chapter Ten, describes shiitake, the delicious culinary mushroom that many believe can help prevent AIDS.

In Chapter Eleven, "Real Stories and Healing Experiences," we allow people who have been touched by medicinal mushrooms to speak. They tell how various mushrooms healed them or changed their outlook on life. Chapter Twelve takes you behind the scenes, where you discover how medicinal mushrooms are cultivated, learn how to shop for medicinal mushroom products, and glimpse some of the people who make the products.

A Note about Scientific Studies from the East

Throughout this book, we present scientific studies on medicinal mushrooms, their immune-modulating properties, and their curative properties. Most of these studies were done in the East, in China, Korea, and Japan. The West has been slow to catch up to the benefits of medicinal mushrooms. Many of the studies that are now being conducted in the West were inspired by studies made in the East.

We believe that the referenced studies conducted in China, Korea, and Japan are valid. They follow the highest standards of scientific protocol. The methods used in the East may vary from those in the West, but the scientists uphold rigorous standards and undertake their studies in the spirit of honest inquiry. They follow sophisticated scientific protocols. The studies we present in this book have been subjected to peer review by panels of international scientists. Some in the West have been quick to criticize scientific data from the East, but we believe that this kind of criticism is unwarranted.

A Word about Taking Medicinal Mushrooms

Finding and working with a healthcare professional who understands alternative medicines is essential if you intend to use unfamiliar treatments. Be sure to let your physician know if you are using an alternative medicine. Your physician can advise you according to your needs and also help monitor the effects of the medicine on your health. Moreover, keeping informed about the latest findings in the health field is essential for your good health. Books like the one you are reading can help lead the way to greater health and vitality.

Scientific research into medicinal mushrooms is still in its infancy. From a medical standpoint, we have only now begun to understand all the benefits of medicinal mushrooms. As more research is conducted, the studies recounted in this book will fade into footnotes. Advances in medical technology will permit research into medicinal mushrooms to go much deeper than it has now. We still have much to learn.

CHAPTER ONE

Introducing Medicinal Mushrooms

IN SEPTEMBER 1991, hikers in the Tyrolean Alps made a remarkable discovery. On a steep, rocky ridge at 10,500 feet above sea level, they found a 5,300-year-old mummy, the oldest intact human being ever discovered. The Iceman, as he came to be known, yielded much information about the neolithic period in which he lived. He carried a copper axe. Previous to the Iceman's discovery, scientists believed that humans were smelting and shaping copper 4,000, not 5,300, years ago. Also, he may have undergone a treatment resembling acupuncture. The tattoos on his legs and back were on or near the acupuncture points for treating arthritis.

To *mycologists*, the botanists who study fungi, the most interesting aspect of the Iceman was his medicine kit. Strung to a leather thong, he carried, two walnut-sized dried fungi that researchers have identified as *Piptoporus betulinus*. The fungus is known for its antibiotic properties. When ingested, it can bring on short bouts of diarrhea. Researchers determined that the Iceman suffered from intestinal parasites. He probably used the *Piptoporus betulinus* in his medicine kit as a natural worm-killer and laxative.

If the Iceman is any proof, neolithic Europeans used mushrooms for their medicinal qualities. Still, as this book will show, the use of medicinal mushrooms in Europe pales when compared with their use in China and Japan. Except in myth and folklore, mushrooms for medicinal purposes were nearly unknown in Western culture. Only in recent years has the West awakened to the medicinal benefits of mushrooms. What accounts for the widespread interest in mushrooms in the East compared to the West?

Mushrooms in Western Culture

Of all cultures, mushrooms are perhaps least valued in the West, especially in regard to their use as medicine. Egyptian hieroglyphics dating to 4,600 years ago show that the pharaohs believed that mushrooms were the plant of immortality. The ancient Egyptians believed that mushrooms growing in the wild were the "sons of the gods" who had been sent to earth on lightning bolts. As such, only the pharaohs were permitted to eat them. The sixteenth-century missionary Bernardino de Sahagún reported that the Aztecs ate a sacred mushroom called *teonanacatl*, which he translated to mean "flesh of the gods." In ancient China, the emperors decreed that all Reishi mushrooms, which were valued as the preeminent tonic herb, be handed over to them (reishi is covered in Chapter Three of this book). Why, then, have mushrooms been neglected in the West?

Until well into the Renaissance, Europeans looked to the ancient Greeks and Romans for their ideas about treating illnesses, and Greek and Roman physicians had little to say about the medicinal qualities of mushrooms. The Roman encyclopedist and naturalist Pliny (23–79 C.E.) described several types of fungi but did so inadequately—it is hard to tell which species he refers to in his writings. The first western pharmacopoeia, *De Materia Medica,* an authority in Europe for 1,600 years, ascribes healing properties to only a single mushroom. Dioscorides (circa 40–90 C.E.), the author of *De Materia Medica,* offers this general description of mushrooms:

> . . . either they are edible, or they are poisonous, and come to be so on many occasions, for either they grow amongst rusty nails or rotten rags, or ye holes of serpents, or amongst trees properly bearing harmful fruits. Such as these have also a viscous concreted humor, but being laid away after they are taken up, they are quickly corrupted growing rotten. But they which are not sod in broth are sweet, yet for all that,

those taken too much do hurt, being hard of digestion, choking or breeding choler.

The Roman philosopher Seneca wrote of mushrooms: "(They) are not really food, but are relished to bully the sated stomach into further eating." Diderot in his *Encyclopédie* wrote, "Whatever dressing one gives to them, to whatever sauce our apiciuses put them, they are not really good but to be sent back to the dung heap where they are born."

The aversion to mushrooms was pronounced in England and Ireland, where the inhabitants as a rule did not eat them or use them as medicine. "Most of them do suffocate and strangle the eater," wrote John Gerard in *The Herball or Generall Historie of Plants*, a compendium of the properties and folkore of plants that was published in 1597.

"Treacherous gratifications," wrote John Farley about mushrooms in *The London Art of Cookery*, published in 1784.

The English physician Tobias Venner wrote about mushrooms in 1620, "Many phantasticall people doe greatly delight to eat of the earthly excrescences called Mushrums. They are convenient for no season, age or temperament." Venner is remembered today as the author of the first tobacco warning label. "Tobacco," he wrote in *Via Recta*, "drieth the brain, dimmeth the sight, vitiateth the smell, hurteth the stomach, destroyeth the concoction, disturbeth the humors and spirits, corrupteth the breath, induceth a trembling of the limbs, exsiccateth the windpipe, lungs, and liver, annoyeth the milt, scorcheth the heart, and causeth the blood to be adjusted."

In "'Mont Blanc'" (written in 1816), a poem that explores the relationship between humankind and nature, Percy Bysshe Shelley paints a vivid picture of mushrooms growing on the forest floor—and he reveals the prejudices of his time and place against mushrooms:

> And plants at whose name the verse feels loath,
> Fill'd the place with a monstrous undergrowth,
> Prickly and pulpous, and blistering, and blue,
> Livid, and starr'd with a lurid dew,
> And agarics, and fungi, with mildew and mould,
> Started like mist from the wet ground cold;
> Pale, fleshy, as if the decaying dead
> With a spirit of growth had been animated.
> Their mass rotted, off them flake by flake,
> Till the thick stalk stuck like a murderer's stake,
> Where rags of loose flesh yet tremble on high,
> Infecting the winds that wander by.

Not all European countries are as mycophobic as the English. In Italy, Poland, and much of Eastern Europe and Russia, mushrooms are an important part of the diet, and the first days of spring find whole families journeying to the countryside to harvest mushrooms. Generally speaking, countries that underwent rapid industrialization are more likely to be mycophobic. In those countries, where industrialization often displaced the rural population, knowledge of native mushrooms and plants is more likely to be lost. In countries with stable rural populations, mushroom lore can be handed from generation to generation as youngsters forage in the company of adults.

Almost everyone is the descendent of immigrants in the United States. For that reason, knowledge of native mushrooms cannot have been handed down in a steady line from one generation to the next. Most Americans are strangers to their mushrooms. That, more than any other reason, explains why Americans are mycophobic. The first and sometimes only thing American children learn about wild mushrooms is that some are poisonous and therefore you should never pick or eat one.

Because mushrooms usually grow in the shadows, in damp places, and in decay; because they look strange and have no counterpart in nature; they were sometimes associated with demons and spirits. The strange excrescences of the forest literally appear overnight—a fantastic occurrence that could only be the work of devils. In medieval times, it was believed that thunder caused mushrooms to sprout in the forest. Many believed that devils and witches used mushrooms to cast spells.

Indeed, the ergot fungus was probably the catalyst for witch trials throughout the Middle Ages, not that the witches' accusers understood why. When the ergot fungus (*Claviceps purpurea*) invades rye and conditions are appropriately damp, peasants who eat the fungus in their rye bread may suffer from ergotism. Because wheat was highly sensitive to diseases, rot, fungal infection, and harsh weather, rye was the grain of choice among the poor masses. Bread was the principle diet in many parts of Europe during the Middle Ages, when people are supposed to have eaten a pound and a half of bread a day, making them especially susceptible to ergotism.

Ergotism causes blisters on the skin, feelings of being pricked, and burning sensations. In extreme cases, sufferers experience convulsions. They have vivid hallucinations. The flow of blood to the limbs is constricted, and limbs may turn gangrenous and fall off. Some scholars blame an outbreak of ergotism for the Salem, Massachusetts, witchcraft trials of 1692. Interestingly, a handful of scholars also argue that ergotism helped launch the Great Awakening of 1741, a religious revival that swept across New England and had participants experiencing visions and trances. In 1943, the Swiss chemist Albert Hoffman, experimenting with ergot alkaloids, discovered LSD.

Two prominent figures of history were killed by mushroom poisoning and their deaths may have contributed to the reputation of the mushroom as a dangerous poison. In 54 C.E., Emperor Claudius of Rome was poisoned by his fourth wife, Agrippina. He is supposed to have died a painful death twelve hours after eating poisonous mushrooms. The Buddha is supposed to have died by a mushroom he believed to be a delicacy. The mushroom was offered as a gift and is said to have been a type that "grew underground," although nothing more is known about it. (However, some scholars believe that the Buddha died from choking on pork, not from eating a poisonous mushroom.) The first known written reference to eating mushrooms is an epigram written by Euripedes in about 450 B.C.E. It tells of a woman and her three children who died from mushroom poisoning.

To be fair to Europeans, mushrooms may have been a part of European medicine in the past. The records are hard to come by because folk medicine was not recorded or valued during the Middle Ages in the same manner as in ancient Greek and Roman medicine. What's more, Christian church officials, operating under the notion that folk healers were pagan practitioners of heathen religions, suppressed folk medicine and sometimes persecuted those who practiced it. Very little research into medicine was recorded during the Middle Ages as the monks busied themselves with copying and recopying Greek and Roman medical texts. Then, with the coming of the Renaissance, European physicians took what they believed to be a more scientific approach to their work. Folk remedies were considered backward and were shunned in favor of contemporary medicines and treatments.

All this is not to say that fungi are not used as medicine in the West. Consider these three important drugs, all of which are derived from fungi:

- Penicillin. Produced from the fungus *Penicillium notatum*, penicillin is one of the most prescribed antibiotics in the world and is routinely used to treat bacterial infections. Thanks to penicillin and other antibiotics, death rates from infectious bacterial diseases are five percent of what they were in 1900.
- Cyclosporin. Produced from two fungi, *Trichoderma polysporum* and *Cylindrocarpon lucidum*, this drug is used in organ transplant operations to depress the immune system and give

transplanted organs a better chance of being accepted by the body. The drug is also used as a treatment for diabetes.

- Krestin. A polysaccharide fraction named PSK, extracted from the *Trametes versicolor* mushroom, is the basis for the pharmaceutical drug Krestin. Before the advent of Taxol, Krestin was the number-one selling anticancer therapy in the world, accounting for hundreds of millions of dollars in sales. Although not approved by the Food and Drug Administration (FDA) in the United States, this drug has a very good track record and a loyal following among oncologists around the world. (Chapter Eight of this book examines the *Trametes versicolor* mushroom.)

As to culinary mushrooms, the prejudice against them may be subsiding in the United States. The bland button mushroom still accounts for the majority of mushroom sales, according to the American Mushroom Institute, but sales of shiitakes, oyster mushrooms, and other more exotic culinary varieties are on the rise. Between 1989 and 1995, sales of shiitake mushrooms doubled. Sales of oyster mushrooms grew by 36 percent. Overall, mushroom sales grew by 25 percent. Black and white morels, porcinis, chanterelles, portobellos, and enokis are now available in some gourmet markets and sometimes in supermarkets as well.

Mushrooms in Western Culture: The Hallucinogens

In recent years, R. Gordon Wasserman, Albert Hoffman, Carl A.P. Ruck, and other scholars have proposed that ancient Greeks and Romans used hallucinogenic mushrooms in their religious rituals. Because the rituals were conducted in private and the participants were sworn to secrecy, the evidence is hard to read. But Wasserman and others make compelling arguments for the use of hallucinogenic mushrooms by Greeks, Romans, and even early Christians.

In Greek mythology, Demeter's daughter Persephone was kidnapped by Pluto, the king of the Underworld. Furious, Demeter killed all the crops, whereupon Zeus, afraid that his subjects would starve and no one would be left to make sacrifices, brokered an arrangement: Persephone would spend a third of the year in Hades with Pluto and the rest of the year above ground with her mother. The myth celebrates birth and regeneration, the return of spring, and the blessings of agriculture.

Annually, the Greeks held a festival in October to commemorate

Demeter's reunion with Persephone. For several days, revelers filled the streets of Athens, and then the festival moved to nearby Eleusis, where a select few were allowed in the initiation hall. There, in the semidarkness, they drank a potion called *kykeon* ("mixture") and beheld the Mysteries of Eleusis. Initiates are supposed to have experienced convulsions and hallucinations. In an anonymous seventh-century B.C.E. poem describing the mysteries, the poet speaks of seeing the beginning and ending of life, a vast circle starting and ending in the same place.

Kykeon was made of barley, water, and mint. Wasserman and his colleagues believe that ergot-infested barley accounts for the hallucinogenic nature of the potion. To back up their theory, they point out that *kykeon* was purple, as is ergot sclerotia when immersed in water. Purple, the color of ergot, was also Demeter's identifying color, and an ear of grain was the symbol of the Eleusinian Mysteries.

We will probably never know whether drinking ergot was a feature of the Eleusinian Mysteries. Nevertheless, it is intriguing to think that Socrates, Plato, and other seminal thinkers of Western philosophy drank ergot, the fungus from which LSD is derived, during the festival of Eleusis.

No less a scholar than Robert Graves has suggested that followers of the Dionysus cult ate the hallucinogenic mushroom *Amanita muscaria* during their autumnal feasts. A mosaic in the ancient Christian basilica of Aquileia in northern Italy clearly shows a basket filled with *Amanita muscaria* mushrooms. Some scholars have suggested that early Christians ate the mushroom in their religious rituals, but the mosaic at Aquileia may well be left over from the original Roman temple, the one from which the basilica was built.

The ritual use of the hallucinogenic mushroom *Amanita muscaria* by shamans and priests in Asia, America, and Africa is well documented. The priests of ancient Europe could well have used the mushroom in their rituals, too. The Vikings are supposed to have eaten it before battle to induce the "berserk" state and make themselves more ferocious to their enemies. The renewed interest in mushrooms in the West has inspired scholars to look into whether ancient Europeans used *Amanita muscaria*, and we look forward to more scholarly research in this area.

The Koryak tribe of Siberia are not Europeans, but their use of *Amanita muscaria* is too interesting not to relate. Filip Johann von Strahlenberg, a Swedish explorer traveling in Siberia in the early 1700s, records how wealthy tribe members assembled in a hut to ingest the mushroom, while the tribe's poorer members, not to be denied the experience, assembled outside. When an intoxicated tribe member left the hut to urinate, those outside gathered around to collect his urine in a bowl so that they could drink and partake of the hallucinogenic mushroom, albeit secondhand.

Medicinal Mushrooms in China and the East

Chinese culture is anything but mycophobic. The prejudice against fungi is entirely absent in China. The Chinese faith in the medicinal qualities of mushrooms is unimpeachable. As anybody who has eaten in a Chinese restaurant knows, mushrooms are a feature of Chinese cuisine. Gathering mushrooms is a popular pastime in the countryside. In China's oldest materia medica, the *Herbal Classic,* many mushrooms are described, so the use of mushrooms for medicinal purposes in China reaches far into the past. (Legend has it that the *Herbal Classic* was written in the twenty-eighth century B.C.E. by emperor Shen Nung, the Divine Plowman Emperor, but most scholars date the book to about 200 C.E.)

Why were (and are) mushrooms valued in the East, but not the West, for their medicinal properties? One can only speculate on this subject, but here are a few possibilities as to why the Chinese value medicinal mushrooms so highly:

- The Chinese never drew a distinction between folk medicine and higher medicine. The physicians who compiled the *Materia Medica* included folk medicines because evidence showed that the medicines prevented disease or cured the sick. In the West, folk medicines were deemed backward and out of date, and they weren't preserved in *Materia Medica.*
- In so far as they traded medical knowledge with one another, Buddhist monks constituted a kind of medical fraternity throughout much of Chinese and Japanese history. The monks, traveling from monastery to monastery, spread information about medicinal mushrooms.
- Taoist priests used medicinal mushrooms in their rituals and for healing purposes. Some aspects of the ancient Chinese religions, including the healing arts, are preserved in Taoism. Therefore, the Chinese never lost their connection to the past and the ways in which ancient people used mushrooms.

- China's legendary bureaucracy helped circulate information about medicinal mushrooms. Most dynasties had a medical official who was responsible for issuing and enforcing health ordinances. The provinces had their medical officials, too, who traded information with one another.

Traditional Chinese Medicine

Throughout this book, we describe how traditional Chinese medicine prescribes mushrooms to treat different ailments. Because most people who read this book are strangers to traditional Chinese medicine, a few words about it are in order.

The traditional Chinese system represents a completely different medical language. It has been said that traditional Chinese medicine attempts to understand the body as an ecosystem or single component in nature. Whereas a Western doctor studies a symptom in order to determine the underlying disease, a Chinese doctor sees the symptom as part of a totality. Western medicine is concerned with isolating diseases in order to treat them. Traditional Chinese medicine seeks a "pattern of disharmony," or imbalance, in the patient.

The principles of traditional Chinese medicine can be found in Taoism, the ancient philosophy or religion in which the practitioner strives to follow the correct path, or Tao, and thereby find a rightful place in the universe. Taoists believe that the universe is animated by an omnipresent life-energy called *Qi* (pronounced CHEE). *Qi*, meanwhile, comprises two primal opposites, *yin* and *yang*. The yin and yang complement each other and are always interacting. They produce change in the universe. They counterbalance each other. Yin, the negative balance, represents water, quiet, substance, and night, among other things. Yang, the positive balance, represents fire, noise, function, day, and other entities. The interplay of yin and yang keeps the universe alive and vital.

In a healthy human body, Qi circulates unimpeded and the balance of yin and yang is maintained, but an excess of yin or yang or a blockage of Qi can create a pattern of disharmony and render the patient ill. No disease has a cause according to traditional Chinese medicine. Rather, disease is a malevolent configuration of yin-yang forces in the body.

Qi flows through the body in invisible channels called *meridians*. In their diagnoses, acupuncturists examine the body's meridian points, the places where Qi is concentrated. If they discover that the body's Qi is congested or needs redirecting, they insert a pin in the proper meridian point.

In keeping with the Taoist idea that the body is a small-scale representation of the cosmos, much of the medical terminology is based on the workings of nature. Physicians examine patients for dampness, wind, cold, dryness, and summer heat. As nature is organized into five primal powers (water, fire, wood, earth, and metal), the body is regulated by five organ networks (kidney, heart, spleen, liver, and lung), each with its own yin-yang energy.

Traditional Chinese medicine encompasses four different ways of treating the sick:

- *Acupuncture.* In acupuncture, stainless steel, gold, or silver needles are applied to the meridian points of the body. Originally, there were 365 acupuncture points, but that number has grown to two thousand in modern times. Most acupuncturists work with 125 or so points, and a typical treatment requires inserting ten to fifteen needles.
- *Moxibustion.* This is the application of burning substances on the meridian points of the body. Mugwort (*Artemisia vulgaris*) is usually the *moxa,* or heating substance.
- *Herbal medicine.*In herbal medicine, herbs and combinations of herbs, including mushrooms, are prescribed to affect the body and bring it into balance. Medical literature describes more than 25,000 formulas—combinations of herbs—that physicians may prescribe for their patients.
- *Tui Na,* or *acupressure.* This involves the massaging and manipulating of the meridian points of the body. The massage techniques are meant to stimulate Qi energy.

Entering into the thought-system of traditional Chinese medicine is not easy for a Westerner. The terminology can be baffling. The system takes ideas and principles that are foreign to Western thought as its premise. To explain the success of traditional Chinese medicine in healing the sick and preventing illness, some in the West dismiss Chinese medicine by crediting its success to the placebo effect. Others take the opposite tack and see traditional Chinese medicine as a sort of faith-based religion. They believe that Chinese medicine, because it is ancient and has roots in the East, is more spiritual and therefore more beneficial than Western medicine.

But traditional Chinese medicine *is* medicine. However strange it may appear to Westerners, traditional Chinese medicine represents the culmination of four thousand years of clinical practice and observation. Like Western medicine, traditional Chinese medicine is an ever-evolving attempt to understand how the body works, how disease affects the body, and how to treat and prevent illness. Although the underlying philosophy is different from Western medicine, the perception of health and illness that traditional Chinese medicine upholds is valid and true to itself.

After the Chinese revolution of 1949, the communist government considered abandoning traditional Chinese medicine. The idea was to embrace Western medicine as part of the campaign to modernize China. Some in the government considered the Chinese brand of medicine backward, a remnant of underdevelopment. To see whether traditional Chinese medicine had any value, the government sponsored numerous clinical studies and tests starting in the 1950s (some of these tests were the first undertaken on medicinal mushrooms). The government's conclusion: Traditional Chinese medicine works clinically and should be given equal footing with Western medicine.

Acupuncture, the most popular brand of traditional Chinese medicine in the West, received a big boost in the United States in 1971 when *New York Times* reporter James Reston, accompanying Secretary of State Henry Kissinger on a trip to Beijing, needed an emergency appendectomy. Reston was treated for postoperative pain with acupuncture, a much-publicized event that put the spotlight on acupuncture as a means of relieving pain. (The focus on acupuncture as an analgesia and anesthetic continues; the clinical benefits of acupuncture are not as well understood or appreciated in the West.) Wrote Reston:

> In brief summary, the facts are that with the assistance of eleven of the leading medial specialists in Peking (Beijing), who were asked by Premier Chou En-lai to cooperate on the case, Prof. Wu Wei-jan of the Anti-Imperialist Hospital's surgical staff removed my appendix on July 17 after a normal injection of xylocaine and benzocaine, which anesthetized the middle of my body.
>
> There were no complications, nausea, or vomiting. I was conscious throughout, followed the instructions of Professor Wu as translated to me by Ma Yu-chen of the Chinese Foreign Ministry during the operation, and was back in my bedroom in the hospital in two and a half hours.
>
> However, I was in considerable discomfort if not pain during the second night after the operation, and Li Chang-yuan, doctor of

acupuncture at the hospital, with my approval, inserted three long thin needles into the outer part of my right elbow and below my knees and manipulated them in order to stimulate the intestine and relieve the pressure and distension of the stomach.

That sent ripples of pain racing through my limbs and, at least, had the effect of diverting my attention from the distress in my stomach. Meanwhile, Doctor Li lit two pieces of an herb called *ai*, which looked like the burning stumps of a broken cheap cigar, and held them close to my abdomen while occasionally twirling the needles into action.

All this took about twenty minutes, during which I remember thinking that it was a rather complicated way to get rid of gas in the stomach, but there was noticeable relaxation of the pressure and distension within an hour and no recurrence of the problem thereafter.

Practitioners of traditional Chinese medicine are now found in most major cities in the West, and not just in the Chinatowns of major cities, either. Nearly thirty American states license or certify acupuncture practitioners. In the United States, approximately 10,000 nationally certified acupuncturists were practicing in the year 1995. Over five million Americans visited acupuncturists in 1997.

As the interest in preventative medicine, natural medicine, and non-drug therapies increases, so does the interest in traditional Chinese medicine. Colleges for its study have been established in France, the United States, Italy, and Australia. In Germany, the University of Münich sponsors an institute for the study of traditional Chinese medicine. This kind of cross-cultural scholarship is bound to open new doors and yield many exciting discoveries.

Fungi and Mushrooms in Nature

What we call a "mushroom" is the *fruit-body* of a fungus. In other words, the mushroom is the reproductive part of the fungus that grows above ground and releases *spores*, the seedlike elements from which new fungi are made. Much as fruit is the reproductive organ of a fruit tree, a mushroom is the reproductive organ of a fungus. Not all fungi, however, produce mushrooms. Some are able to create spores and reproduce without bearing a fruit-body. Fungi that reproduce without a sexual stage are called imperfect fungi, or *fungi imperfecti.*

In nature, fungi are the great recyclers. To feed itself, but also to assist plants in getting the nutrients they need, a fungus breaks down organic matter into essential elements. There are about a hundred thousand species of fungi and 38,000 mushroom species. About seven hundred species are eaten as food. Fifty or so species are poisonous. Fungi make up about a quarter of the biomass of the earth. Strange as it may seem, seeing as they are usually associated with rot and decay, fungi are something of a cleanser in that they transform dead organic matter into nutrients that plants and animals can feed on. Without fungi, matter would not break down and decompose. The world would be crowded with dead animals and plants. The odor from so much unregenerated decay would be dreadful.

Every fungus begins as a tiny, seedlike spore. Spores are carried by wind and water. When a spore lands in a hospitable place—a moist place that is not too hot or cold and is near a food source—it may germinate and start a new fungus colony. At that point, the spore grows *hyphae,* the fine, threadlike strands from which the mycelium is made.

The *mycelium* is the feeding body of the mushroom. Composed of a latticework of interconnected hyphae threads, it is for the most part subterranean, living in soil or decayed wood, much like the root system of a plant. It can feed on almost any organic *substrate:* soil, wood rot, food left for too long in the pantry. How fast and how large the mycelium grows depends on environmental factors such as soil temperature and the accessibility of food. Researchers have reported finding a mycelium beneath the soil of Michigan that is 1,500 years old and thirty-five acres wide, and weighs a hundred tons. This mycelium is from the fungus *Armillaria bulbosa*, a root pathogen of Aspen. Using molecular methods, the researchers mapped the extent of the fungus genome to show that the mycelium germinated from a single spore. In case you're in the neighborhood, the researchers place the monster on the upper peninsula of Michigan at 45°58'28" N longitude, 88° 21'46" W.

The mycelium insinuates itself into the substrate on which it feeds. It secretes complex enzymes that break down organic material in such a way that the fungus can absorb food from the substrate. Research has shown that these complex enzymes act as a growth stimulus to plants. They degrade organic material so that important nutrients are returned to the soil where plants can feed on them. In this way, fungi provide the raw material for trees and plants.

Fungi are essential for a healthy forest. If there are no fungi in the soil, plants cannot grow as they cannot break down and absorb nutrients without the help of fungi. One group of mushrooms, called the *mycorrhizae,* attach themselves to the roots of trees. They act like a secondary root system, reaching deep into the soil to get nutrients that the tree could not otherwise get and passing these nutrients upward to the tree. In return, trees provide the mycorrhizal fungus with a set of nutrients that they need to grow. The fungus and tree work together in a symbiotic partnership.

In effect, fungi are molecular disassemblers. They take the complex compounds created by plants, such as cellulose, carbohydrates, and protein, and disassemble those compounds so that plants can digest them. By contrast, plants are molecular assemblers. They take very simple compounds such as water, nitrogen, and carbon and combine them into complex forms such as protein, carbohydrates, and cellulose.

Some scientists believe that the ability of fungi to break down organic matter is linked to the antidisease properties of fungi. Fungi live in a hostile environment amongst decay on the harshest layer of the ecosystem. There, they encounter disease-causing pathogens far more frequently than other life-forms. To survive, they must have proactive, healthy immune systems. Some scientists believe that the antipathogen properties in mushrooms are precisely what make mushrooms valuable to the human immune system.

To ensure its survival, every fungus produces spores, the incredibly light agents of fungal reproduction. In most fungi, spores are produced in the fruit-body, the mushroom part of the fungi that grows above the soil. Typically, spores sprout from the *gills,* the thin brown tissue found on the underside of the cap. Borne by the wind, some kinds of spores are capable of traveling great distances from the fruit-body to start their own fungus colonies.

Mushrooms produce prodigious numbers of spores. A giant puffball, for example, may produce 20 trillion. The spores are produced in such large numbers to guarantee the spread of the fungus in the environment. The mycologist Elio Schaechter has written about spores, "Lavishness is necessary; rare is the spore that germinates into successful fungal growth. Such wastefulness, however, is not unlike the production of millions of unsuccessful sperm cells by the human male."

Are Fungi Intelligent?

Fungi, in their own small way, may exhibit a primitive intelligence. How else can one explain advanced behavior on the part of certain fungi? To make the case for fungi being intelligent, we present *Cordyceps curculionum* and the amoebalike slime mold *Physarum polycephalum.*

Cordyceps refers to different varieties of fungi that grow and feed on the bodies of insects. (Chapter Four of this book describes *Cordyceps sinensis,* a mushroom that grows from the bodies of caterpillars in the mountains of China and Nepal.) In the case of *Cordyceps curculionum,* the spore attaches itself to an ant, germinates, begins feeding, and grows into a small mushroom. The ant, meanwhile, with the mushroom riding piggyback, goes about its normal business. One day, however, the ant is seized with a sudden desire to climb a tree, and up it goes. When it reaches a height sufficient for the release of the *Cordyceps curculionum* spores, the ant digs its mandibles into the tree and remains there for the rest of its life. When it finally dies, the spores are released from on high and are spread far and wide on the forest floor. *Cordyceps curculionum* shows admirable restraint by not eating the ant right away. Its display of moderation in the presence of food seems to demonstrate a level of intelligence that isn't present in a few people we know.

To test the intelligence of the slime mold *Physarum polycephalum,* Toshiyuki Nakagaki of the Bio-Mimetic Control Research Center in Nagoya, Japan, placed pieces of the mold in the middle of a five-square-inch maze. In the two exit points of the maze, he placed a food source, ground oat flakes. The idea was to see whether the fungus would abandon its normal method of foraging for food—by spreading outward from a central point of germination—and instead grow directly toward the food sources. To his surprise, Nakagaki discovered that the mold did indeed go straight toward the food sources. The organism stretched itself in a thin line along the contours of the maze until it reached the exit points. Similar to a laboratory rat, the slime mold was able to negotiate the maze and find the source of food.

By navigating the maze, *Physarum polycephalum* demonstrated a kind of intelligence that is not usually found, for example, at shopping malls. Mall shoppers are known to wander aimlessly in the shopping maze until they arrive by accident at the thing they want. *Physarum polycephalum* knows how to get there straightaway.

CHAPTER TWO

Strengthening the Immune System with Medicinal Mushrooms

THROUGHOUT THIS BOOK, we describe how medicinal mushrooms can promote good health. Mushrooms strengthen the immune system. They contain substances such as terpenoids and beta glucan that awaken the immune system and give it a boost. Mushrooms have a beneficiary effect on prebiotics in the gastrointestinal tract. They are adaptogens, substances that help the body adapt during times of stress.

Beta glucan, terpenoids, prebiotics, adaptogens—are these terms unfamiliar? They are explained in this chapter. This chapter provides the scientific background for the rest of the book. Here, you will find descriptions of the medical processes and medical terminology that pertain to medicinal mushrooms. We wrote this chapter to help you make wise decisions when it comes to taking medicinal mushrooms and other health supplements.

An Alert, Awake Immune System: Medicinal Mushrooms as Immunoregulators

Problems in the immune system come in two varieties. When the immune system is underactive, it makes you susceptible to infections and cancer.

When it is overactive, it may create allergies and autoimmune reactions. *Autoimmune* means the immune system is overstimulated and mistakenly attacks the body. Diseases such as diabetes, lupus, and lymphoma are autoimmunity diseases. AIDS, hepatitis, the flu, and colds, on the other hand, are associated with a weakened, underactive immune system.

As more research is conducted on medicinal mushrooms, it has become evident that some of them are immunoregulators. An *immunoregulator* is any substance that can quiet or activate the immune system, depending on circumstances. An immunoregulator quiets an overactive immune system; it increases activity when the immune system is sluggish. Basically, an immunoregulator triggers the production of white blood cells when the system is underactive, and it lowers their number when the system is overactive.

The optimal immune system is alert and ready to battle disease, but it is not overactive. An overactive immune system can cause autoimmune disorders such as allergies and create trouble of its own. As immunoregulators, medicinal mushrooms can help the body attain an optimal immune system. Mushrooms can help the immune system stay wide awake and strike the perfect balance between overactivity and sluggishness.

Importance of a Strong Immune System

Many physicians believe that a greater emphasis on strengthening the immune system is overdue. Rather than concentrate all their efforts on treating disease, these physicians believe in teaching their patients to prevent disease as well. A good diet, getting the right amount of exercise, managing stress, and getting enough sleep all strengthen the immune system. Another practical way to fortify the immune system is to include medicinal mushroom products in your diet. Medicinal mushrooms have a proven effect on macrophages, T cells, and other important agents of the immune system.

Statistics such as these, which pertain to people in the United States, underscore the need to maintain a strong immune system:

- One of three Americans will get cancer in his or her lifetime.
- There are 1.2 million new cases of cancer each year in the United States.
- Six million Americans suffer from seasonal allergies, a disorder brought about when the immune system overreacts.

· Forty million Americans suffer from heart disease (caused initially by an inflammatory process).

· Ninety thousand Americans die each year from infections they acquired in hospitals. Two million suffer from such infections annually (hospitals create "superbugs," and hospitalized people are weak and therefore more susceptible to disease).

Compromised immune systems have also given rise to lasting disorders such as diabetes, eczema, irritable bowel syndrome, chronic fatigue syndrome, and Epstein-Barr disease. By some estimates, as much as seventy percent of the United States' health care budget is devoted to treating people with chronic ailments. About a third of the people who suffer from them can't go to work or attend school.

In order to understand all the different ways that medicinal mushrooms can help strengthen the immune system, a little background is necessary. The next handful of pages outlines the immune system and its major components.

How the Immune System Works

In the course of a single day, the body may encounter billions upon billions of bacteria, microbes, viruses, parasites, and toxins. When you get a cut or an insect bite, bacteria and viruses enter your body. When you draw a breath, bacteria and viruses enter your lungs. When you take a bite of food, millions of germs enter your digestive tract. How the immune system handles these invaders is extremely complex and there is much that we don't know. The immune system's network of organs, cells, and molecules reaches into almost every part of the body.

One way to grasp the workings of the immune system is to think of the immune system as a country. Like a country, the immune system has border guards whose duty is to provide protection from outsiders. It has customs officials who check incoming cells and microorganisms to determine whether they should be admitted. If an unwanted invader penetrates the border, the immune system can mount a counterattack with its army of white blood cells. The immune system's intelligence agency keeps dossiers on undesirable bacteria and viruses so it can recognize and destroy those elements when they arrive. The immune system also has mechanisms for handling civil wars and rebellions. If the immune system is overstimulated, it can harm the body, but the system's civil guards can quiet revolts and maintain the peace. All the agencies work together to make sure that the immune system is a healthy, well-functioning entity.

Self-Tolerance: Knowing Which Cells Belong in the Body

The central duty of the immune system is to distinguish between what belongs to the body and what doesn't belong. For this reason, every cell that originates in the body has distinctive molecules—identification papers, so to speak—that mark it as belonging. Immune system cells do not attack cells that have their papers in order. However, all cells that originate outside the body are suspect. Foreign cells have distinctive molecules called *epitopes*. When the immune system encounters a foreign cell that it recognizes and knows to be harmful, it takes steps to halt the invader. These invaders are known as *antigens*. An antigen can be a bacterium, virus, microbe, parasite, or toxin. An antigen is any substance that provokes the immune system to act. The ability of the immune system to distinguish between cells that belong to the body and cells that don't belong to the body is called *self-tolerance.*

Guarding the Surfaces of the Body

The first line of defense against disease—the border guards, so to speak—is the skin and mucus membranes. The skin wraps the body and creates a boundary between the body and the outside world. It secretes antibacterial substances that kill off most bacteria as soon as they arrive. The mucus membranes protect the nose and mouth against germs. Mucus contains an enzyme called lysozyme that breaks down bacteria before they can do any harm.

Lymphatic System: The Army of the Immune System

The lymphatic system comprises a network of lymph nodes whose purpose is to filter out and drain contaminants and bacterial infections from the body. There are about six hundred lymph nodes, or glands, most of them clustered around the neck, groin, and armpits. The system carries *lymph*—a fluid composed chiefly of white blood cells called *lymphocytes*—from the tissues to the bloodstream. As lymph flows through the body, it filters the body of disease. During an examination, doctors often feel the lymph nodes in the neck to see if they are swollen. Swollen lymph nodes mean that the nodes are producing additional white blood cells because the body is fighting an infection.

Cells of the Immune System

The cells of the immune system, to stretch a metaphor a bit farther than perhaps it should be stretched, are like the police. They patrol the different parts of the body and attack invaders or spread information about invaders. The cells that become immune cells originate in the bone marrow, primarily in the legs, from stem cells. From there, the cells can develop into a number of different types. In brief, here are the different kinds of immune cells:

- T cells. One kind of T cell, the *helper T cell,* identifies invader cells with a chemical marker so that they can be destroyed by other cells (the HIV virus destroys helper T cells). Another kind of T cell, called the *cytotoxic T cell,* destroys cells that have been infected by viruses or mutated by cancer. Still other T cells suppress the activity of the immune system when it gets overstimulated.
- Cytokines. These are messengers that alert the immune system to the presence of an invader. T cells, B cells, and macrophages secrete cytokines. Cytokines are the alarm signal of the immune system. They tell the immune system to be on the lookout for invaders.
- Natural killer cells. These hungry cells travel in the bloodstream looking for foreign cells. When they find a foreign-invader cell, they destroy it.
- B cells. These cells secrete antibodies. The antibodies bind to and destroy antigens. There are many kinds of B cells and each is programmed to produce a certain kind of antibody that kills a certain kind of antigen.
- Phagocytes (monocytes, neutrophils, and macrophages). This category refers to the very large white blood cells that can engulf and destroy invaders. Monocytes circulate in the blood; macrophages circulate in the tissue; neutrophils are found in the blood but can move into the tissues if they are needed there.

The macrophage, a particularly powerful cell, deserves special attention because it plays an important role in boosting the immune system. What's more, as you will learn later in this chapter, medicinal mushrooms are known to have a stimulating effect on macrophages.

Macrophages were discovered in the 1880s by Dr. Elie Metchnikoff, a Russian biologist. Noting their size and ability to devour other cells, he created the term *macrophage* from the Greek *macro,* which means "big," and *phage,* which means "eater." Metchnikoff used the term *phagocytosis* to describe the process by which the macrophage destroys the foreign invader.

As soon as a macrophage encounters a foreign organism or substance, it engulfs and destroys it with a barrage of cell-killing enzymes. Macrophages, along with other cells such as dendritic cells, are antigen-presenting and antigen-processing cells, or APCs. These cells present a harmless fraction of the antigen they have just destroyed to T cells so that T cells can learn what the antigen is and be able to recognize and attack it themselves. Next, the macrophage secretes cytokines, the cell messengers that alert the immune system to the presence of an invader. The result is a "chemical frenzy" or "immune cascade" in which natural killer cells and T cells are produced in large numbers to repel invaders. So, besides killing antigens on its own, a macrophage plays a key role in recognizing when the body is being attacked and alerting the body to an attack.

Antibodies and Immunoglobulins

Each type of antibody is programmed to bind to and possibly neutralize a certain kind of antigen. Antibodies are secreted by B cells. When a B cell encounters an antigen with which it is familiar, it produces large plasma cells, and these cells, in turn, produce antibodies in large numbers. The antibodies go out and bind to the antigen. In effect, the B cell makes the prototype antibody for attaching to an antigen, and the plasma cell takes the prototype and creates many antibodies from it.

Antibodies are members of a family of large protein molecules called *immunoglobulins.* There are nine types of immunoglobulins. Some serve to help other cells in the immune system kill microorganisms. Others activate cells of the immune system, such as B cells. Some kill bacteria. One class, IgE, is involved in the defense against parasites, but because most parasites are under control in the urban population of the United States, IgE is also associated with allergies in most Americans.

The Immune System's Memory

Like the nervous system, the immune system can build a memory. When T cells and B cells are activated to fight a disease, some become memory cells. These cells store information about the disease and pass it on to the next generation of cells. In this way, the immune system can recognize bacteria and viruses it has confronted before and stop them. Throughout our lives, the immune system adds to its memory of microbes, bacteria, and viruses, and it becomes more competent at fighting disease.

The Rise and Decline of the Immune System

Incidences of cancer are on the rise. We see higher rates of heart disease and diabetes. More people suffer from allergies. According to some, there is a worldwide asthma epidemic. In Australia, for example, two of every five primary school students have been diagnosed with asthma.

Some people read the reports about higher disease rates and conclude that pollutants and toxins are to blame. According to these people, synthetic compounds in the air and water, emulsifiers and preservatives in processed food, and the depletion of the ozone layer have weakened the immune system. These people—and some of them are quite shrill—think that the immune system is under siege. They believe that modern life with its peculiar stresses and environmental challenges has put the immune system on trial and made the body more susceptible to disease.

Rates of disease *are* rising, but we believe that the cause has less to do with environmental factors and more to do with improvements in medical science. Improvements in medicine, paradoxically, have led to an increase in disease. Advances in medicine have helped push life expectancies past age seventy-five in most industrialized countries. The older you are, however, the weaker your immune system becomes, and the more likely you are to acquire an illness. As the number of older people rises, so do incidences of disease. What's more, from the point of view of genetics, adults on average have weaker immune systems than they did in the past. In times past, to put it crudely, the natural selection process in the form of diseases such as infectious diarrhea, measles, and whooping cough weeded out children with weak immune systems and unfit genomes. Most of these children died in the first year of life.

As adults, the children who would have died in earlier times from a childhood disease are more likely to be ill because their immune systems are weaker. This combination of an older population and a weaker immune system in the average adult has caused the rise in disease rates.

From what we know of records kept in Western Europe and North America (the only regions where reliable records were kept), life expectancy in the mid-eighteenth century was between thirty-five and forty-two years. Cancer was essentially unknown because most cancers occur after the age of fifty. Many diseases were ignored in spite of the efforts of anatomists and anatomo-pathologists who started working during the eighteenth century when the ban on dissection and autopsies was lifted. Tumors were considered accidents of nature. Indeed, the era produced beautifully illustrated medical textbooks with pictures of tumors, and one could see models of tumors in the wax museums of Europe, but tumors were merely a curiosity. Menopause was totally unknown because not enough women reached the age of menopause.

The nineteenth century saw real improvements in medicine. Edward Jenner administered the first immunizations against smallpox around 1800. Joseph Lister developed his antiseptic surgical techniques in 1865. Louis Pasteur identified germs at about the same time. By 1900, these medical discoveries and others pushed life expectancies in industrialized countries to about age fifty-five. Diseases such as cancer and diabetes were still not well known or understood. The dread disease of the nineteenth century, the disease whose name evoked fear and anxiety the way *cancer* does in our day, was tuberculosis. People still did not live long enough to acquire cancer in great numbers, although the disease did receive attention. Physicians believed, and rightfully so, that cancer was rare in people younger than forty. One physician observed that cancer was most likely to occur in people who live in temperate climates in the "highest state of culture and civilization," but that it was entirely absent in Native Americans and infrequent in African Americans. We may presume, given the conditions under which they lived in the nineteenth century, that these groups rarely lived long enough to get cancer in significant numbers.

In the past hundred years, life expectancy has jumped in most industrialized countries past seventy-five years of age. Moreover, the natural selection process by which children with weak immune systems died in the first year of life has ended. Is it any wonder that diseases that thrive on a weakened immune system—allergies, cancer, asthma, diabetes, and heart disease—are on the rise? If a polluted environment were the cause of rising rates of disease, incidences of asthma would be decreasing, not increasing, for example, in Los Angeles and Denver. Starting about 1975, those cities embarked on ambitious plans to curb air pollution. They succeeded by every measure in spite of population growth. The air over Denver and Los Angeles has seen a reduction in particulates due to diesel fuel, nitrogen oxide, and sulfur dioxide. Nevertheless, asthma rates have risen in Los Angeles and Denver. They have risen because asthma is an inflammatory disease often associated with allergies and the extra production of IgE, a disease more likely to occur in people who have a weak or compromised immune system. Asthma is brought about by various cells of the immune system that appear to go into overdrive and remain in a chronically activated state. The result is a chronic inflammatory disorder of the airways that results in their narrowing and makes breathing extremely difficult.

The immune system begins developing during the first weeks of gestation. The cell-mediated immunity that is associated with T cells develops in the womb. The fetus has an immune response very, very early in life. When a child is born, he or she has a fully intact natural immune system. The system is stimulated after birth and reaches its peak at the onset of puberty, between age eleven and fifteen (sometimes later if and when children live in a hygienic environment). At that time, the immune system reaches a plateau; starting at age thirty-five or so, it doesn't work as well. Some parts of the immune system work well, but others are lazy, and others work too well and perhaps cause autoimmune disorders.

After age 50, the immune system experiences a decline. To be blunt, the human body is not supposed to live past that age. Nature, cruel and pitiless, wants you to make room for subsequent generations after your fiftieth birthday. However, advances in medical science, agriculture, and social organization have pushed life expectancies past age seventy-five in some countries.

A Look at Some Diseases of the Immune System

Diseases of the immune system are more likely to arise when the immune system is underactive or overactive. As we mentioned at the start of this chapter, an optimal immune system is well balanced. It is neither sluggish nor overstimulated. When the immune system is underactive, the body is more likely to get colds, the flu, and even cancer. An overstimulated immune system makes the body more susceptible to autoimmune or allergic disorders such as diabetes, asthma, and allergies. The following pages look at diseases of the immune system so you can get a better idea of how the immune response works.

Autoimmune Diseases

Autoimmune refers to what happens when the immune system attacks itself. Getting back to our metaphor of the immune system as a country, an autoimmune disorder occurs when civil war erupts and members of the army engage in insurrection. In an autoimmune disorder, the immune system has trouble distinguishing which cells rightfully belong in the body and which do not and it mistakenly attacks cells of the body.

Diabetes is an autoimmune disorder. It is caused by abnormally high blood sugar levels. Either the body doesn't produce insulin or it isn't able to use insulin effectively. For reasons that are not fully understood, immune-system cells mistakenly attack the beta cells in the pancreas that produce insulin and the result is an autoimmune reaction. Macrophages, the huge white blood cells that attack foreign cells, attack the beta cells, and this inspires the T cells to get into the act. They mark the beta cells as enemies, and soon the entire immune system attacks the beta cells. Now the beta cells cannot regulate the amount of sugar in the bloodstream and the result is a sugar buildup. Several medicinal mushrooms have proven themselves effective against diabetes. These mushrooms have been known to quiet the immune system when it is undergoing an autoimmune reaction.

Lupus, known as *systemic lupus erythematosus,* or SLE, is another autoimmune disease. Effective treatments are still lacking and the cause is unknown. The disease gets its name from the red patch that often appears on the forehead of sufferers that resembles a V-shape, like the dark patch on the forehead of a wolf (the wolf's Latin name is *lupus*). The symptoms vary greatly and can include rashes, inflammation of the fluid membrane surrounding the lungs, arthritis, anemia, rashes, seizures, oral ulcers, and low white blood cell counts. Many lupus patients have signs of fatigue, anxiety, or depression. The disease is treated with immunosuppressants, steroids, and nonsteroidal anti-inflammatory drugs.

An allergy is also a disease involving the immune system's going into overdrive. Allergies are associated with antibodies of a class called IgE. When someone who is prone to allergies encounters an allergen for the first time, the person's B cells produce large numbers of antibodies of the type that are designed to counteract the allergen. The antibodies attach themselves to mast cells in the nose, tongue, skin, and gastrointestinal tract. The next time the person encounters the allergen, the mast cells produce chemicals that cause sneezing, watery eyes, and other symptoms of an allergic reaction.

There are practically no allergies to mushrooms. In fact, by being immunoregulators, mushrooms seem to help some people decrease the frequency and the intensity of their allergic reactions. According to some good but limited reports, mushrooms appear to decease the allergic component of the immune response.

Diseases Caused by an Impaired or Sluggish Immune System

Cancer is a complex disease that can affect any organ or system of the body. Causes of the disease include genetic defects, uncontrollable cell growth, and cell damage caused by radiation or toxins. In some respects, cancer is a natural occurrence in the body. According to a recent study, six detectable tumors are produced each year in the body of the average American. If you went to the doctor every day of the year and were probed in the right locations, you would be diagnosed with cancer six times. In most people, however, the immune system eradicates cancerous tumors before they become a health issue.

With approximately 100 million cells dividing in the body per day, some replications are bound to occur in error. One job of the immune system is to identify and destroy these aberrant cell replications before they can divide and pass on their aberrations. When the immune system doesn't recognize that a dividing cell is aberrant, the cell can continue to grow, and the immune system may not be able to treat it if it grows too large. The result is cancer.

By way of their polysaccharides, medicinal mushrooms stimulate natural killer cells, cytotoxic T cells, and the macrophages to look for tumor markers on the surface of malignant cells, identify these cells, and destroy them. Medicinal mushrooms help the immune system work better and be more alert, especially at an early age. In effect, medicinal mushrooms tell the cells that patrol the body for abnormalities—the soldiers in the barracks, so to speak—to get up, start circulating, and do their jobs better.

AIDS is caused by the *human immunodeficiency virus,* or HIV. The virus progressively destroys the body's lymphocytes, the white blood cells that circulate in the lymph nodes and flush viruses and bacteria from the body. The disease has a particularly damaging effect on the helper T cells that mark antigens in the body so they can be destroyed. Because antigens such as bacteria and parasites are not marked, they are able to infiltrate and damage the body.

Understanding Polysaccharides and Beta Glucan

When we eat plants and mushrooms, we digest the polysaccharide molecules and they enter our systems. One type of polysaccharide is called beta glucan. Many researchers believe that beta glucan is what gives some mushrooms their medicinal properties. The following pages explain polysaccharides and beta glucan.

Introducing Polysaccharides and Beta Glucan

Mushrooms and plants are composed of *polysaccharides,* which are long chain molecules constructed from sugar units (*poly* means "many," *saccharide* means "sugar"). How the polysaccharides arrange themselves into structural units and how they bind together determine what compounds they form. For example, *cellulose,* the cell wall material in plants, represents a particular configuration of polysaccharides. *Chitin,* the cell wall material in mushrooms (as well as insects, shrimp, and sponges), represents a different configuration.

Beta glucan molecules, or simply beta glucan (or β-glucan), are one configuration of polysaccharide. As you will see, beta glucans are found in abundance in medicinal mushrooms and are one reason why medicinal mushrooms strengthen the immune system. The term *beta glucan* refers to the way that the sugar units are attached to one another in the polysaccharide chain. Each glucose molecule has six carbons. For that reason, the linkage between the different carbons can occur at any combination of six positions. A polysaccharide in which the molecule at the first position is linked to the next molecule at the third position is called a 1-3 beta glucan. Most beta glucan in mushrooms is of the 1-3 variety and is known to boost the immune system. Plants, by contrast to mushrooms, mostly contain 1-4 beta glucan in which the molecule at the first position is linked to the next molecule at the fourth position.

A beta glucan is a huge molecule. To see how large, consider penicillin, which is one of the largest molecules at 500 or more molecular weight. Compounds found in plants can sometimes reach 45,000 or 50,000 molecular weight. The beta glucan molecules found in mushrooms, however, are typically 1.5 to 2 million molecular weight. Mushroom beta glucan is a whole order of magnitude more complex than other molecules. The size of mushroom beta glucans has a lot to do with their value as immune-system stimulators, although the size and complexity of beta glucan molecules also make it hard for scientists to study precisely why they are so beneficial to the immune system.

One problem with taking beta glucan as a health supplement is that, due to the size of the molecules, beta glucan can be difficult to digest. However, beta glucans are chain molecules. Like any other chain, they can be broken down, and one segment of the chain has all the properties of the other segments. Vitamin C has been known to help the digestive system break down beta glucan.

How Beta Glucan Aids the Immune System

Beta glucan does not in and of itself cure disease. It makes the immune system work better so that diseases can be prevented from attacking the body. No one knows precisely how beta glucan stimulates the immune system. Beta glucan molecules are so large, it is hard for scientists to trace their action in the body. Nevertheless, it appears that beta glucan molecules resemble the molecules found on bacterial cell walls. In effect, beta glucan molecules are phantoms that make the body believe it is being invaded by a bacterium. When macrophages—the giant white blood cells that guard the body against disease—encounter a beta glucan, they believe that they have encountered a bacterium and they attack. This gives a boost to the entire immune system. Immune cells, such as T cells, are put on alert. Levels of immunoglobins (in other words, antibodies) increase. The immune system believes it is under attack and it goes into a state of high alert. It takes all the measures it normally takes when it detects the presence of a virus, bacterium, or tumor cell.

The unique molecular shape of beta glucan permits it to bind to certain receptor cells on the surface of macrophages and other kinds of white blood cells. In effect, the beta glucan molecule puts its key into the macrophage and unlocks it. As a result, free radicals are produced. Free radicals are molecules that have one or more one unpaired electron. As the section entitled "Mushrooms and Free Radicals" explains later in this chapter, free radicals help kill bacteria, viruses, parasites, and malignant cells, although they can also damage normal cells and their production must be controlled.

Within macrophages, beta glucan has also been shown to stimulate the production of cytokines, the cell messengers that tell the immune system when it is being attacked. Cytokines aid macrophages in stopping the growth of and destroying tumors.

To test the health benefits of beta glucan, scientists at the laboratories of Alpha-Beta Technology in Worcester, Massachusetts, incubated beta glucan in blood and examined the results. They discovered that beta glucan indeed caused free radicals to appear in white blood cells. Beta glucan also stimulated the growth of megakaryocyte and myeloid progenitor cells. These types of cells develop into immune cells.

Each mushroom appears to produce its own slightly different type of beta glucan. The length of branching along the glucose chain differs in the beta glucan found in different mushrooms. For that reason, each mushroom stimulates the immune system in a slightly different way. Because each glucose molecule has six carbons, glucan chains that are thousands of units long can join in a nearly infinite number of ways, and the different beta glucan structural arrangements have a similar but slightly different activity in the body.

In the next decade, as scientists focus their attention on the immune-enhancing properties of beta glucan, we are sure to learn more about the different varieties and how they prevent disease. For now, we know that the beta glucans from the maitake mushroom, for example, stimulate the production of T cells. *Agaricus blazei,* on the other hand, has a very unique 1-6, bonded-chain beta glucan. The mushroom offers almost no T cell stimulation activity, but it stimulates the production of natural killer cells.

The United States Food and Drug Administration (FDA) has granted GRAS (Generally Recognized As Safe) status to beta glucan. It can be extracted from other substances besides mushrooms, notably from algae, oats, wheat, and brewer's yeast. Medicinal mushrooms, however, offer the greatest variety of beta glucan. What's more, medicinal mushroom products offer more than just beta glucan. They also offer antibacterial and antiviral compounds.

Beta Glucan Studies

Interest in beta glucan as a health supplement began in the 1940s when scientists working under Dr. Louis Pillemer extracted a crude substance they called Zymosan from the cell walls of yeast. Dr. Pillemer and his colleagues understood that the substance activated the immune system, but they didn't know how or why. In the 1960s, Nicholas DiLuzio of Tulane University succeeded in isolating 1-3 beta glucan as the active component of Zymosan. Wrote Dr. DiLuzio, "The broad spectrum on immunopharmacological activities of glucan includes not only the modification of certain bacterial, fungal, viral, and parasitic infections, but also inhibition of tumor growth."

In the 1980s, Dr. Joyce Czop of Harvard University unraveled the mystery of how beta glucan stimulates immunity. She observed a 1-3 beta glucan docking to receptor sites on the surface of a macrophage cell and determined that this docking activity stimulated the macrophage to action. She wrote, "Beta glucans are pharmacologic agents that rapidly enhance the host resistance to a variety of biologic insults through mechanisms involving macrophage activation."

One of the first clinical experiments with beta glucan occurred in 1975 when Dr. Peter Mansell of the National Cancer Institute attempted to see whether beta glucan could aid in the treatment of malignant melanoma, a dangerous form of skin cancer. Dr. Mansell injected beta glucan into the nodules of the skin cancer in nine patients. He wrote that the cancer lesions were "strikingly reduced in as short a period as five days" and, in small regions, "resolution was complete."

Interestingly, one of the first large-scale tests of beta glucan was conducted on fish. In the 1980s, the Norwegian salmon-farming industry was hit with huge losses due to bacterial infections in the fish. The salmon were fed antibiotics, but the bacteria soon produced resistant strains and the antibiotics proved ineffective. One scientist, Dr. Jan Raa of the University of Norway, decided to try a novel technique. He introduced beta glucan into the food supply, and the infections soon disappeared.

Over the past two decades, the number of scientific studies on beta glucan has been growing steadily (in 1996, there were 144 scientific studies in all). Here are a handful of revealing trials and studies on the immune-enhancing effects of beta glucan:

· In a double-blind, placebo-controlled clinical trial conducted under Dr. William Browder of Tulane University, twenty-one patients who had undergone high-risk gastrointestinal surgery were given beta glucan intravenously each day for a week. Dr. Browder and his colleagues wanted to find out if beta glucan could boost the patients' immune systems and reduce post-operative infections. Only nine percent rate of the patients who received beta glucan contracted infections, a figure considerably lower than the forty-nine percent in patients who did not receive beta glucan. What's more, the mortality rate among those who received beta glucan was zero, whereas the other patients who had undergone surgery for physical trauma suffered a twenty-nine percent mortality rate.

- Scientists at Tulane University School of Medicine injected beta glucan directly into the chest-wall malignant ulcers of women who had received mastectomies and radiation from breast cancer. The ulcer sores healed completely.

- In a study undertaken at Zhejiang University in Hangzhou, China, a beta glucan concentrate derived from maitake mushrooms was administered to lung-cancer patients who had undergone chemotherapy. Patients who received the concentrate as well as the chemotherapy had higher survival rates than patients who received only the chemotherapy.

- To test the effect of beta glucan on fungal infections, scientists at the State University of São Paulo in Brazil gave conventional antifungal drugs to two test groups, one comprising eight and one comprising nine patients. The nine-patient group also received beta glucan intravenously for one month. Thereafter, the group was given monthly doses for eleven months. At the end of a year, the group that had received beta glucan did not have a single relapse, whereas the other group experienced five relapses. Members of the beta glucan group also had lower traces of fungal infection in their blood.

Beta Glucan and Cholesterol

Beta glucan has a demonstrated ability to lower cholesterol levels. The United States Department of Agriculture (USDA) conducted a study to determine if adding beta glucans to the diet lowers cholesterol levels. Twenty-three volunteers suffering from high cholesterol took part in the study. In the first week, all were put on a diet in which 0.8 percent of their calories came from beta glucans and thirty-five percent came from fat. Starting in the second week, one group of volunteers received an oat extract with one percent beta glucan, and another group received an oat extract with ten percent beta glucan. After three weeks, when the study concluded, cholesterol levels in the group that received the larger amount of beta glucan dropped significantly. Cholesterol levels dropped in the other group as well, but not as dramatically. Researchers are not certain why beta glucan lowers cholesterol levels. One theory is that beta glucan traps bile acids—which were made from cholesterol—and flushes them from the body. As bile acids leave the body, cholesterol does too. Another theory is that beta glucan decreases the production of cholesterol by the liver.

Beta Glucan and Asthma

Asthma is a chronic inflammatory disorder that causes the airways in the lungs and throat to narrow. The narrowing can be caused by pollutants, smoke, pollen, dust, or other stimuli. Five percent of the population of the United States is supposed to suffer from asthma. Interestingly, asthma rates are higher in industrialized countries than developing countries. Some physicians believe that the high rates of asthma in industrialized countries are caused by the relative cleanliness of those countries. These physicians believe that the body, especially in childhood, needs to be exposed to mycobacteria, viruses, and parasites so that it can learn to fight off microbes. People in developing countries, these physicians argue, do not contract asthma as often because their bodies have learned to counteract mycobacteria.

One theory is that beta glucan can help prevent asthma because beta glucan molecules are similar in shape to those of mycobacteria. The theory is that asthma sufferers and people who are susceptible to asthma can use beta glucan as a substitute for mycobacteria. In so doing, they can build up the The cell response that prevents asthma.

Absence of 1-3 Beta Glucan in the Modern Diet

As we have demonstrated, 1-3 beta glucan helps the body build a strong immune system. Beta glucan stimulates the production and activity of T cells, natural killer cells, and macrophages. Some scientists believe that cancer, arthritis, allergies, and other diseases that result from a weakened immune system are on the rise because people are not getting enough 1-3 beta glucan in their diet. Processed foods and so-called fast foods are probably to blame.

As we explained earlier, plants mostly contain 1-4 beta glucan, but plants contain a small amount of 1-3 beta glucan —the kind found in mushrooms—as well. Oats and wheat have the highest 1-3 beta glucan levels. In these grains, as much as two or three percent of the molecules are 1-3 beta glucans. In the past, most people obtained their 1-3 beta glucan from grains such as oats and wheat, but the amount of 1-3 beta glucan in those grains has dropped in recent years. Modern food-processing companies prefer grains with low 1-3 beta glucan levels. These grains contain less fiber. They are easier for people to digest. Animals who eat corn and oats with low levels of 1-3 beta glucan absorb the grains better and do not produce as much dung (a useless byproduct on the modern farm, where chemical instead of natural fertilizers are used). Because modern food-processing companies prefer grains with less fiber (and less 1-3 beta glucan), farmers grow those grains. The result is a loss of 1-3 beta glucan in the modern diet, a loss for which you can compensate by making medicinal mushrooms a part of your diet.

Medicinal Mushrooms as Adaptogens

The term *adaptogen* was coined in the 1940s by a scientist of the defunct Soviet Union named Dr. Nicolai Lazerev. In his studies of wild Siberian ginseng, Dr. Lazerev noticed that the herb had a quieting affect on the nervous system and helped reduce the effects of stress on the body. Dr. Lazerev used the term *adaptogen* to describe herbs like ginseng that help the body adapt during times of stress. Two colleagues of Dr. Lazerev, I. I. Brekhman and I. V. Dardymov, refined the definition of an adaptogen as follows: "[It] must be innocuous and cause minimal disorders in the physiological functions of an organism, it must have a nonspecific action, and it usually has a normalizing action irrespective of the direction of the pathological state." In traditional Chinese medicine, adaptogenic herbs and medicines are usually termed *tonics*. A tonic herb is one that makes the body more resilient and strengthens the body's natural defenses.

Scientists are discovering that stress engages many different areas of the body: the nervous system, the cardiovascular system, hormone production, and others. The problem, some scientists believe, is that the body's response to stress was conditioned in prehistoric times when humankind faced acute, short-term, life-threatening stress, not the long-term, persistent stress and anxiety we face today. When the body experiences stress, the adrenal glands secrete hormones, the sympathetic nervous system quickly arouses itself, the heart beats faster, blood pressure rises, and the amount of sugar in the blood increases. Some scientists believe that the body often overreacts to stress. Sustained periods of stress can tax the nervous system and cardiovascular system. They can disrupt hormone production. Long-term stress can lead to cardiovascular disease, fatigue, and depression. The cumulative effect of all this may result in a weakened immune system.

Consider, for example, the effect of increased cortisol levels in the body. To help cope with stress, the adrenal glands produce increased amounts of a hormone called cortisol. Increases in cortisol are normal when faced with a life-threatening situation. For example, the adrenal glands secrete higher levels of cortisol to reduce unnecessary and painful inflammation and thereby heal wounds. However, long-term increased levels of cortisol can cause diabetes and fatigue, as well as weaken the immune system.

Adaptogens are believed to let the adrenal glands recharge, stabilize the body's hormone production, and help the body control blood sugar levels. Many herbs are considered to have adaptogenic properties, including different varieties of ginseng, astragalus, and licorice root. Three mushrooms described in this book—reishi, shiitake, and maitake—are considered adaptogens.

Terpenoids in Mushrooms

Many medicinal mushrooms contain terpenoids. *Terpenoids* help the immune system and the healing process in various ways. Generally speaking, they are good at killing bacteria and viruses. They are anti-infectious agents. Some terpenoids protect the arteries of the heart. Many of them are anti-inflammatory. This means that they prevent the immune system from overreacting.

The word *terpenoid* comes from the *turp* in *turpentine.* Turpentine, made from the resin of pine trees, has been used as an antiseptic for cleaning wounds and cuts since the time of the ancient Greeks. When scientists studying turpentine isolated the substance that gives turpentine its healing power, they coined the word *terpenoid* to describe the substance. Terpenoids are found throughout nature, not just in turpentine. Like turpentine, many substances and plants that contain terpenoids give off a slightly bitter aromatic odor.

The anti-inflammatory role of terpenoids is especially valuable to the healing process. To see why, consider what happens when you get a cold. The cold virus causes the nose and throat to swell and redness to appear around the nostrils and nose. The swelling and the redness are part of the inflammatory process due to reactions of the immune system. The immune system sends white blood cells to attack the infection, and as more white blood cells arrive, the area around the infection starts swelling. Sometimes, however, there is too much swelling and an inflammatory reaction occurs. In the case of a cold, the inflammatory process exceeds it goals and creates an inflammation that is useless for the patient. The nose and throat constrict and breathing becomes difficult.

An inflammatory reaction in the arteries can have especially bad consequences. In this case, the wall of the artery can swell and encumber the flow of blood. Many physicians believe that heart disease is caused initially by an inflammatory reaction in the arteries. This is why many doctors recommend aspirin to patients. Aspirin, like the terpenoids, is anti-inflammatory. Steroids such as cortisone are also anti-inflammatory. The inflammation that accompanies an infection is healthy as long as it is kept under control. To control inflammation, if necessary, we can use anti-inflammatory substances, but many of these substances also block the benefits of the immune response. Cortisone, for example, prevents inflammation but also allows germs to proliferate.

The beauty of terpenoids is that they temper the action of the immune system's response to infections. They are anti-inflammatory, but not to the extent that they prevent the white blood cells from doing their job. Terpenoids respect the natural healing process while protecting against inflammation. They stimulate the body's immune defenses, kill germs, prevent inflammation, and give the patient a degree of comfort. By the way, terpenoids are some of the oldest medications. To cure the common cold, people have been inhaling the fresh resin of pine trees and eucalyptus leaves for many, many years. Pine tree resin and eucalyptus leaves both contain terpenoids.

Medicinal Mushrooms and Prebiotics

You may be interested to know that there are ten thousand times more germs in your gastrointestinal tract than there are cells in your body. By some estimates, bacteria in the large intestine account for ninety-five percent of all cells in the body. Most people carry around three to four pounds of bacteria in their gastrointestinal tract. These germs amount to a sort of ecosystem that is different in the body of each individual. Some of the bacteria are good and some may be bad. Bifido bacteria, for example, prevent diarrhea and constipation. Pathogenic *E. coli*, on the other hand, causes severe cramps, diarrhea, and sometimes death. Due to diet, viral infections, bacterial infections, or the use of antibiotics, normal bacteria in the intestinal tract can be depleted. When this happens, pathogenic bacteria may predominate and cause an illness.

Prebiotics are substances that help the good bacteria in the intestinal tract. They are a sort of intestinal fertilizer in that they promote the growth of beneficial bacteria. Prebiotics feed microorganisms that are helpful to the intestinal tract, and they kill microorganisms that are not helpful. They produce vitamins of the B family. They assist the body in absorbing minerals such as calcium and magnesium. Prebiotics aid the immune system by killing pathogens. Some researchers believe that they also lower blood cholesterol, prevent diarrhea, and help fend off colon cancer.

High-fiber foods such as mushrooms are prebiotics. These foods help bacteria in the large intestine to breed in a balanced, harmonious way. Mushrooms are a class above many other prebiotics because they contain terpenoids that are antimicrobial but don't affect the good germs in the intestinal tract. Mushrooms also stimulate M cells in the lining of the intestine. These cells, similar to antigen-presenting and APCs, kill antigens and microbes but also pass along samples of the antigens and microbes they have killed to the immune system. In this way, the immune system is awakened and put on alert for invaders.

By the way, be careful not to confuse prebiotics with probiotics. A *probiotic* is a live bacterial culture like that found in yogurt and other fermented dairy products. Probiotics are also good for the intestinal tract. They provide bacteria that the intestinal tract needs to stay healthy.

Mushrooms and Free Radicals

A *free radical* is an atom of oxygen whose composition is the same as that of bleach. As everyone knows, bleach is used in the household to kill bacteria—and it is used the same way in the body. To kill bacteria, viruses, parasites, and malignant cells, white blood cells and macrophages release free radicals. However, if these free radicals proliferate too freely, they may kill normal cells. As a result, body tissue dies—in muscles, bones, skin, and elsewhere—and the body ages faster.

In biochemistry, substances called *antioxidants* are capable to a certain extent of reversing the damage that free radicals do to body tissue. Mushrooms are antioxidants. Perhaps the three most well-known antioxidants are vitamin C, vitamin E, and beta-carotene. Taking antioxidants helps reduce unnecessary free radicals. By bringing the number of free radicals to a normal, more acceptable level, antioxidants control the aging process.

However, some antioxidants can have a harmful effect on the body. In a recent study conducted in Finland, beta-carotene supplements were given to smokers who had contracted lung cancer. Smoking encourages the production of free radicals in the lungs. The body, to kill the toxins that smoking brings in, produces free radicals, but these free radicals can kill normal cells and thereby kill normal tissue as well. The researchers in Finland wanted to see if taking the synthetic antioxidant beta-carotene would curb the production of free radicals in the smokers' lungs. They were puzzled to discover that beta-carotene had the opposite effect: more free radicals were seen in the smokers' lungs. This study and others like it seem to show that beta-carotene actually encourages the production of free radicals in the stressed parts of the body in which there is already an excess of free radicals. In other words, taking the antioxidant beta-carotene can be harmful in some instances.

Antioxidants can also be harmful if you exceed the optimal dosage. Studies indicate, for example, that taking too much vitamin C actually encourages unnecessary free radicals to be released in the body. This is why the National Academy of Sciences recommends taking no more than one gram per day of vitamin C.

The good news for people who make mushrooms a part of their diet is that it you never run the risk of stimulating the unnecessary production of free radicals. Mushrooms do not produce excess free radicals anywhere in the body. As to exceeding the optimal dosage, it is hard to do that with mushrooms. You will experience indigestion and bloating long before you reach the optimal dose.

Protective Effect on the Liver

The liver is the body's second largest organ (the skin is its largest). The job of the liver is to detoxify the body. The liver is the body's chemical plant. It manufactures cholesterol, which every membrane of every cell needs. The liver produces approximately twenty proteins, including antibodies and the proteins that are involved in the inflammatory process by which the immune system attacks infections. These proteins ensure that the body fights infections without going to excessive lengths. If the liver doesn't function well, the inflammatory process is impaired.

It appears that some substances in mushrooms have a protective effect on the liver. Mushrooms have been used to treat a variety of liver disorders, including hepatitis, a disease that infects 350 million people, according to the World Heath Organization. In a study of 355 cases of hepatitis B treated with the Wulingdan pill, which includes the fruit-body of the reishi mushroom (Chapter Three describes reishi), 92.4 percent of the subjects showed positive results. Lentinan, the drug derived from *Lentinula edodes* (the shiitake mushroom described in Chapter Ten), has shown favorable results in treating chronic persistent hepatitis and viral hepatitis B. *Trametes versicolor* (the subject of Chapter Eight) is sometimes prescribed for chronic active hepatitis and hepatitis B.

The Trouble with Antibiotics

To better understand the value of maintaining a strong immune system, consider how antibiotics such as penicillin have been used and abused by doctors and their patients. When antibiotics were introduced in the 1940s, they were presented to the public as a kind of miracle drug. And antibiotics have performed many miracles. Death by infectious bacterial disease is five percent of what it was a hundred years ago. In 1900, hospitals were very dangerous places. If bacteria entered and infected a surgical incision, the patient often died.

The trouble with antibiotics, however, is that bacteria find ways to fight and resist them. Some bacteria are very resilient. As they fight off antibiotics, they develop into new strains—strains that are sometimes resistant to antibiotics. The dilemma is caused by natural selection. The antibiotic kills most bacteria, but the strongest survive and hand down their survival characteristics to the next generation. Some bacteria train plasmids to convey the resistance to other bacterial species. In effect, antibiotics have created new diseases.

Consider the bacterium *Streptococcus pneumoniae*. The bacterium causes pneumonia and meningitis. Each year, it causes half a million cases of pneumonia and an estimated seven to ten million ear infections in children. Doctors used to be able to treat the bacteria with penicillin, but some strains of the bacteria have become resistant to antibiotics.

"This super-bacteria explosion is a public health crisis of the first order," reports Dr. Jack Dillenberg, Director of the Arizona Department of Health Services. "If left unchecked, we face potentially devastating consequences, including widespread sickness and death from once-curable diseases."

Ironically, doctors are forced to prescribe antibiotics more frequently as the drugs become less potent. By some estimates, 190 million doses of antibiotics are administered each day in hospitals—that's right, *each day*. Annually, doctors prescribe more than 130 million courses—doses administered over a few days or weeks—to their out-of-hospital patients. The numbers are alarming. They underline the importance of preventing disease by maintaining a healthy immune system. Take the following precautions with antibiotics to make sure you use them wisely:

- Do not overuse antibiotics. A sickness is also an opportunity for the immune system to test itself and grow stronger. If you take antibiotics at the first sign of infection, you weaken your immune system in the long run.
- Take the full course of treatment, even if you believe that you have been cured. If you stop taking the drugs midway through the treatment, you will kill all but the most virulent bacteria, which will remain in your system.
- Don't skip a dose. Doing so allows the bacteria in your system to rest and grow stronger.
- Follow the doctor's instructions for taking the antibiotic.
- Don't take antibiotics for flus or colds. These diseases are caused by viruses, and antibiotics do not work against viruses.
- Do not treat yourself with old antibiotics from the medicine cabinet.
- Do not use soaps with antibacterial chemicals unless you are ill with a bacterial disease.

Why Not Get Mushrooms in the Supermarket?

Some of the mushrooms that are described in this book can be purchased in gourmet markets and supermarkets. That begs the question, "Can culinary mushrooms provide the same health benefits as medicinal mushroom products?"

Culinary mushrooms are an aid to health. They appear to be a good source of B vitamins, iron, niacin, riboflavin, thiamine, and ascorbic acid. By proportion to weight, mushrooms are high in polyunsaturated fats. Cultivated varieties contain large amounts of carbohydrates and fiber. On a dry-weight basis, a mushroom is high in protein, and mushroom proteins contain essential amino acids.

The relationship between good health and a diet rich in mushrooms came to the attention of modern science when health researchers noticed that people who eat mushrooms seem to be healthier than other people. In Japan, for example, scientists discovered fewer incidences of cancer in shiitake-growing regions (shiitake is described in Chapter Ten of this book). Assuming that people who lived in these regions ate the shiitake mushroom often, scientists wanted to see whether shiitake had anticancer properties. They ran many tests on shiitake. In so doing, they discovered and introduced Lentinan, the third most widely prescribed anticancer drug in the world.

Some mushrooms are better than others. Shiitake, for example, stimulates the immune system about a hundred times more than the common white button mushroom does. Maitake (described in Chapter Six of this book) does much more to aid the immune system than do morels, portobellos, chanterelles, or any other culinary mushroom. Still, all mushrooms are excellent for your heath. The difference between culinary mushrooms and medicinal mushrooms is that medicinal mushrooms are a class above their culinary cousins.

Taking a mushroom product in capsule or powder form has distinct advantages because most mushroom products are made from the mycelium, the feeding body of the mushroom that grows underground. Mycelium is a potent substance. You could say that mycelium is nature's way of concentrating the beneficial compounds of mushrooms. When you buy a culinary mushroom, however, you buy the fruit-body. Fruit-bodies do not always contain the potent concentrations of polysaccharides that are found in mycelium. (Mycologists are currently perfecting cultivation techniques whereby the fruit-body of mushrooms can contain potent concentrations of polysaccharides.)

What's more, medicinal mushroom products are more hygienic. The mycelium powder is subjected to autoclave sterilization before it is pressed into pills or poured into capsules. Taking medicinal mushrooms in pills or capsules is easier on the digestive system, too. The mycelium finds its way into the body faster than the fruit-bodies of mushrooms do.

Because nonorganic, storebought mushrooms are often sprayed with pesticides, eating them regularly may actually be harmful. For that reason, we recommend buying culinary mushrooms at health food stores and other places where organic products are sold.

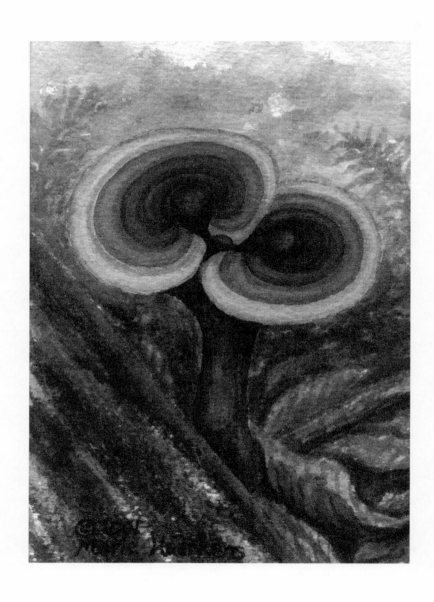

CHAPTER 3

Reishi Mushroom

The Mushroom of Immortality

THE NAMES BY WHICH reishi is known give an idea of how revered the mushroom is in China and Japan. To the ancient Chinese, the mushroom was called *lingzhi*, or "spirit plant" (alternate spellings are *ling zhi, ling qi,* and *ling chi*). The Chinese character for *lingzhi* is composed of three pictures, one for "shaman," one for "praying for," and one for "rain." Reishi has been called the "ten-thousand-year mushroom" and the "mushroom of immortality" because it is said to promote longevity. Reishi, the name by which it is known in the West, comes from the Japanese. The mushroom is also called the "varnished conk" on account of its shiny appearance, and the "phantom mushroom" because it is so scarce in the wild. The mushroom's Latin name is *Ganoderma lucidum,* the etymology of which is as follows: *gan* means shiny, *derm* means skin, and *lucidum* means brilliant. Reishi has been called the king of herbal medicines, with many herbalists ranking it above ginseng. The late Professor Hiroshi Hikino of the University of Tohoku in Japan, a premier authority on Eastern medicinal plants, called reishi "one of the most important elixirs in the Orient."

Reishi is not a culinary mushroom. Although some people use reishi to brew teas, the mushroom is usually taken for medicinal purposes as it has a very bitter, woody taste. Reishi is bitter because the mushroom contains terpenoids, the aromatic substances that have been known to have an anti-inflammatory effect (Chapter Two explains terpenoids). However, the cultured mycelium of the mushroom is not bitter, so people who take it in powder or capsule form need not be bothered by a bitter flavor.

Modern herbalists use reishi to treat a variety of ailments, including chronic fatigue syndrome and diabetes. It is believed to detoxify the liver and help cure hepatitis. Reishi can lower cholesterol, prevent the growth of tumors, and prevent blood clots. In traditional Chinese medicine, reishi is used to treat asthma, gastric ulcers, insomnia, arthritis, and bronchitis. The mushroom is supposed to be an antihistamine and has been known to ease the suffering associated with bronchial asthma and hay fever. Reishi is also used to alleviate the symptoms associated with stress.

Reishi is considered a tonic. As such, it can build energy and increase stamina, although many herbalists warn that it works as a sedative in the short term. It is believed that vitamin C assists the body in absorbing reishi. For that reason, many doctors and herbalists recommend taking vitamin C along with the mushroom.

Reishi in the Wild

In its natural habitat, the reishi mushroom is found in the dense, humid coastal provinces of China, where it favors the decaying stumps of chestnut, oak, and other broad-leaf trees. In Japan, it is usually found on old plum trees. The mushroom's most distinguishing feature is its shiny, lacquered look. Reishi's lustrous, well-preserved appearance may have contributed to its reputation as an herb that promotes longevity. It has a kidney-shaped cap that does not rot or lose its shape after drying. Sometimes the spores appear on the cap and give the appearance of sandpaper. The mushroom comes in six colors: red (*akashiba*), white (*shiroshiba*), black (*kuroshiba*), blue (*aoshiba*), yellow (*kishiba*), and purple (*murasakishiba*). Mycologist Malcolm Clark speculates that these mushrooms will be separated by taxonomists into different species in the next ten to twenty years because the morphology of the mushrooms is different. Red reishi is the *Ganoderma lucidum*, the mushroom that is used for medicinal purposes and is the subject of this chapter.

The reishi mushroom is extremely rare and difficult to find in the wild. Because the husks of the spores are very hard, the spores can't germinate as readily as the spores of other mushrooms. To germinate, the right combination of oxygen and moisture conditions is needed. Fortunately, mycologists are now able to recreate favorable growth conditions in the laboratory (Chapter Twelve describes some advanced growing techniques). The mushroom that was once the provenance of the emperors of China can now be purchased in health food stores.

Folklore of Reishi

Reishi, like most of the mushrooms that are described in this book, has a colorful past. According to legend, Taoist priests in the first century c.e. were the first to experiment with reishi. They are supposed to have included the mushroom in magic potions that granted longevity, eternal youth, and immortality. The Taoist priests of the period practiced alchemy, and they were known for casting spells and mixing concoctions. They were looked upon as magicians or wizards. By present-day standards, these Taoists might be considered charlatans, but we must be careful not to look upon them with disdain or prejudice. Remember that alchemy is the beginning of chemistry. In wizardry begins science. Shamans, who treat the sick by summoning the forces of nature to the aid of their patients, were the first doctors. A poem by the first-century philosopher Wang Chung remarks on the Taoist priests' use of mushrooms in their quest to attain a higher state of consciousness:

> They dose themselves with the germ of gold and jade
> And eat the finest fruit of the purple polypore fungus
> By eating what is germinal, their bodies are lightened
> And they are capable of spiritual transcendence

Reishi achieved pride of place in China's oldest materia medica, the *Herbal Classic*, compiled about 200 c.e. In characteristic Chinese fashion, the *Herbal Classic* divides the 365 ingredients it describes into three grades: superior, average, and fair. In the superior grade, reishi is given first place, ahead of ginseng. To qualify for the superior grade, an ingredient must have potent medicinal qualities and also produce no ill effects or side effects when taken over a long period of time. The book says of reishi:

> The taste is bitter, its atmospheric energy is neutral; it has no toxicity.
> It cures the accumulation of pathogenic factors in the chest. It is good

for the Qi of the head, including mental activities. It tonifies the spleen, increases wisdom, improves memory so that you won't forget. Long-term consumption will lighten your body, you will never become old. It lengthens years. It has spiritual power, and it develops spirit so that you become a "spirit-being" like the immortals.

Reishi's reputation as the "mushroom of immortality" reached Emperor Ti of the Chin Dynasty about twenty-three centuries ago. The Emperor is supposed to have outfitted a fleet of ships manned by three hundred strong men and three hundred beautiful women to sail to the East, where reishi was believed to be growing, and bring back the mushroom. The ships were lost at sea. Legend has it that the shipwrecked castaways washed ashore on an island and founded a new nation there. The island, the story goes, is called Japan.

In the *Pen T'sao Kang Mu* ("The Great Pharmacopoeia"), a sixteenth, century text, compiler Le Shih-chen had this to say about reishi: "It positively affects the life-energy, or Qi of the heart, repairing the chest area and benefiting those with a knotted and tight chest. Taken over a long period of time, agility of the body will not cease, and the years are lengthened to those of the Immortal Fairies."

The Reishi Mushroom in Chinese Art

In Chinese art, the reishi mushroom is a symbol of good health and long life. Depictions of the reishi mushroom can be found on doors and door lintels, archways, and railings throughout the Emperor's residences in the Forbidden City and the Summer Palace. At various times in Chinese history, the Emperor's official scepter included a carving of a reishi mushroom. One emperor's silk robe shows a peach tree, cloud forms, and, prominently, a reishi mushroom.

To the general population, the image of Reishi appears to have been a good luck charm or talisman. In pen and ink drawings, tapestries, and paintings, subjects sometimes wear jewelry or jade pieces made in the image of the reishi mushroom. Kuan Yin, the Chinese goddess of healing and mercy, is sometimes depicted holding a reishi mushroom.

Some believe that the resurrection plant in the popular fairy tale "White Snake" is the reishi mushroom. In the fairy tale, known to all Chinese children and the subject of operas and song, Lady White travels to faraway Kunlun Mountain to obtain the resurrection plant and revive her deceased husband. By demonstrating her love for her husband, she wins the plant, and her husband is revived.

Recent Studies of Reishi

Reishi has been part of the Chinese pharmacopoeia for many centuries. Knowing its reputation as a healing herb, scientists began studying reishi in earnest beginning in the 1980s. In the following pages, we present some of the most up-to-date studies on reishi.

Reishi and Skin Cancer

Aging doesn't damage the skin; sunlight does. Sunlight is not just light and warmth. It is also composed of ultraviolet light. This kind of light can penetrate the skin and cause all kinds of damage to blood cells, nerves, and even the eyes. Long periods of exposure to ultraviolet light can damage the skin's DNA. When the DNA is damaged and cannot recover, it may degenerate, and the result can be skin cancer.

To see if reishi can prevent this kind of damage and skin cancer as well, Korean scientists isolated DNA, placed it in vitro in a hot-water extract of the mushroom, and exposed it to ultraviolet radiation. They concluded that reishi shows "radioprotective ability" and guards against DNA damage. The experiment seems to indicate that eating reishi can slow the aging of the skin and protect as well against skin cancer.

Avoiding the ultraviolet rays of the sun is nearly impossible, but we can take precautions to keep exposure to a minimum. Wearing a hat and covering the skin helps. Applying sunscreen to the skin is also advisable, although only sunscreens that guard against ultraviolet A and ultraviolet B light are of real value.

Reishi and the Effects of Radiation Therapy

Sometimes cancer patients are prescribed radiation therapy. The purpose of the therapy is to kill cancer cells. However, radiation can have harmful side effects. Radiation—and sunlight as well, if you are exposed to it for too long—damages DNA. It has a hindering effect on the ability of blood cells to reproduce and proliferate. Radiation also kills blood cells, including the white blood cells that travel the bloodstream and go to infected areas.

White blood cells are produced in the bone marrow. The part of the bone marrow that produces white blood cells is very sensitive to radiation. As a result, one consequence of radiation therapy is a reduction in the number of white blood cells that are produced. Having fewer white blood cells can be dangerous because it makes the body more susceptible to infection and disease.

To test whether reishi can aid cancer patients who have undergone radiation, scientists at Hebei Academy of Medical Sciences in Shijiazhuang, China, did an experiment on laboratory mice. They irradiated the mice and then fed them spores from the reishi mushroom. The results of the experiment showed that reishi prevents the number of white blood cells from decreasing. Reishi also improved the survival rate of the irradiated mice. The experiment seems to indicate that reishi improves the immune function by keeping the production of white blood cells from dropping in spite of radiation.

Reishi as an Antioxidant

Terpenes, the chemicals found in terpenoids, are known to be anti-inflammatory (terpenoids are explained in Chapter Two). This means that they temper the action of the immune response. When you get a cut, for example, white blood cells assemble at the point of infection and cause swelling and redness. In other words, an inflammation occurs. But if the inflammation grows too big, the healing process is impaired. Terpenoids and other anti-inflammatories keep the inflammatory response in check and prevent it from harming the body.

Recently, scientists at the Chinese University of Hong Kong isolated some substances in reishi that belong to the terpene group. The scientists detected the following fractions: ganodermic acids A, B, C, and D, lucidenic acid B, and ganodermanontriol. These are very powerful antioxidants. An *antioxidant* is any organic substance that is able to counteract the damaging effects of free radicals on body tissues.

Red blood cells carry oxygen and remove carbon dioxide, an essential process for the functioning of the body. However, if the red blood cells do not do their jobs correctly, oxygen can have damaging effects. The antioxidants uncovered in this study help regulate oxygen use.

From this excellent study, we can glimpse how reishi fortifies the body and helps the system stay in balance.

Reishi and Tumors

Essentially, the immune system can fight malignant cancer cells in three ways. One way is for cytotoxic T cells to kill the cancer cells outright. Another way is for the cancer cells to be weakened, and, in their weakened state, for the normal cells of the immune system to kill the cancer cells. The third way is for substances similar to toxins to kill the cancer cells. Three of the toxinlike substances that have been associated with controlling the growth and survival of malignant cancer cells are as follows:

- Tumor necrosis factor alpha, or TNF alpha
- Interleukin 1 beta, or IL-1 beta
- Interleukin 6, or IL-6 (*interleukins* are messenger cells that allow the white cells to communicate with one another)

To examine the immunomodulating and antitumor effects of reishi, scientists in Taiwan isolated polysaccharides from the fruit-bodies and tested them in vitro. The scientists discovered an increase in the production of the three toxinlike substances. The macrophages, monocytes, and T lymphocytes all increased their production of TNF alpha, interleukin 1 beta, and interleukin 6.

Interestingly, the increase in the three substances went to the upper level of the normal range. Too much TNF alpha can kill normal cells, for example, but the reishi polysaccharides did not cause the production of TNF alpha to rise to unsafe heights. This demonstrates the immunomodulating characteristic of reishi. It appears that reishi gives a push to the immune system, but the mushroom doesn't push too far and overstimulate the immune system.

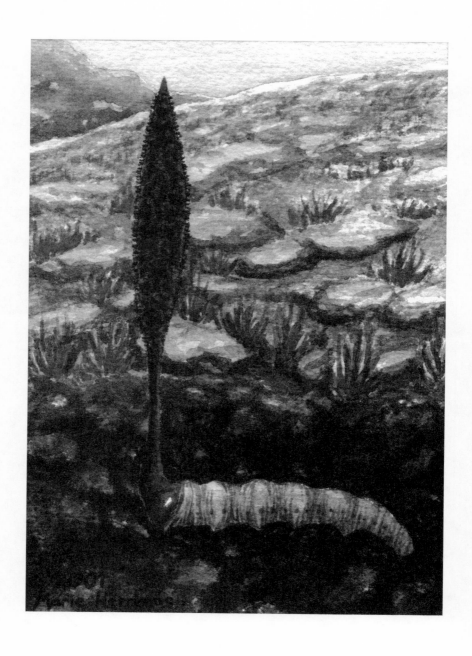

CHAPTER FOUR

Cordyceps Sinensis

The Anti-Aging Mushroom

IN SEPTEMBER 1993, a scandal broke out in the wake of the National Games in Beijing, China. In a single week, three women's track and field world records were broken. Never had a single track meet produced so many world records. Running the 10,000-meter race on Sunday, September 8, the first day of the meet, Junxia Wang shattered the previous world record by an amazing 42 seconds to finish at 29:31.78 (her record still stands). On Tuesday of that week, the record in the 1,500-meter race was broken by Yunxia Qu, who completed the race in 3:50.46, a full three seconds faster than the previous record (Qu's record also stands). On Thursday, when qualifying heats, for the 3,000-meter race were held, giddy fans watched as the world record fell twice, first to Linli Zhang, who broke the record in the first heat, and then again to Junxia Wang, who broke her teammate's newly minted record in the second heat. On Friday, in the 3,000-meter final, the crowd cheered as Junxia Wang broke her own world record by six seconds to finish the race in 8:06.11 (a record that still stands).

Some in the world of track and field cried foul. For so many world records to fall in one place in such a short time, the athletes must have been taking illegal performance-enhancing drugs. Surely, when urine tests were completed, the results would show that the women members of the Chinese national track team had been taking anabolic steroids or some other illegal drug.

But the urine tests came up negative. If the athletes had taken drugs, the tests did not show it. When reporters pressed him to say why his athletes ran so well, Coach Ma Zunren mentioned their rigorous training schedule, their passionate commitment to track and field, and a secret elixir made from the *Cordyceps sinensis* mushroom. (All of Ma's runners had a falling out with their disciplinarian coach and only one made the team that China sent to the 1994 World Track Championships. Ma claims that his runners' performances lapsed because they no longer had access to his secret elixir.)

The wonders of *Cordyceps sinensis* have been known in China for at least a thousand years, where the mushroom is recognized as a national medicinal treasure, a precious and virtually sacred tonic. As a health supplement, it is known to increase energy and vitality. *Cordyceps* is one of the safest medicinal foods. The mushroom is used to treat liver diseases, cancer, angina pectoris, and cardiac arrhythmia. It is prescribed for bronchial problems, anemia, tuberculosis, jaundice, emphysema, infertility, and sexual dysfunction. In traditional Chinese medicine, *Cordyceps* is believed to boost the yang and go to the meridians of the lungs and kidneys, where it acts as an invigorator.

The mushroom has a long and storied history in China. The first mention of *Cordyceps sinensis* appears in 620 C.E. during the Tang Dynasty. The literature describes a strange organism that lives high in the mountains of Tibet and is able to change from animal to plant and back to animal again. That sounds far-fetched, but the ancient literature concerning *Cordyceps* is not as bizarre as it would seem. *Cordyceps sinensis* is indeed an unusual mushroom. It germinates in a living organism, the larvae of certain kinds of moths, chiefly the bat moth (*Hepialus armoricanus*), which it mummifies, colonizes, and eventually kills.

Introducing *Cordyceps Sinensis*

There are over 680 documented varieties of cordyceps mushroom, of which *Cordyceps sinensis* is but one. Many *Cordyceps* fungi besides *Cordyceps sinensis* grow by feeding on insect larvae and sometimes on mature insects.

In appearance, *Cordyceps sinensis* makes for an unusual sight. The mycelium is encased in the mummified body of the caterpillar from which the fungus germinates. The fruit-body, sprouting from the caterpillar, is capless, shaped like a blade or twig, dark brown at the base, and black at the top. Large fruit-bodies sometimes branch out in the manner of antlers (the reason why *Cordyceps* is sometimes called the deer fungus). The mushroom is found at altitudes of nine thousand to fourteen thousand feet. It grows in the alpine meadows of the Himalayas and other high mountain ranges of China, Tibet, and Nepal.

The Latin etymology of *Cordyceps sinensis* is as follows: *cord* means "club," *ceps* means "head," and *sinensis* means "China." The mushroom is also called the "caterpillar fungus" on account of its origin, and, less frequently, the "winter worm, summer plant" because the ancient Chinese believed that the fungus was an animal in winter and a vegetable in summertime. Around 1850, Japanese herbalists began importing the mushroom from China. They named it *tochukaso,* a Japanese translation of "winter worm, summer plant." The mushroom is sometimes called the club-head fungus, a direct translation of its Latin name. The common name used in China today is *dong chong xia cao,* or *chong cao* for short.

There are actually many varieties of *Cordyceps* in nature. *Cordyceps* grow on just about every category of insect—crickets, cockroaches, bees, centipedes, black beetles, and ants, to name a few. Chapter One of this book describes how *Cordyceps curculionum* attacks the body of ants and rides the ants high into the trees to disperse its spores.

Folklore of *Cordyceps Sinensis*

When spring arrives and the snow starts melting in the high mountains, the indigenous people of Tibet and Nepal, as they have done for centuries, take their yak herds to grazing lands at higher elevations. Arriving in the high country, the yaks feed on the fresh spring grass. They paw the ground and remaining snow to expose and eat the *Cordyceps* mushroom. Then, in a frenzy, they begin rutting. As the story goes, herdsmen who observed the yaks rutting in a fever pitch wondered what gave the animals their vitality. Did they eat some kind of animal aphrodisiac? The herdsmen wondered how the animals managed to conduct themselves so vigorously in spite of the high elevation, and they wondered if what was good for the yak might be good for them.

Upon close examination, the herdsmen discovered that the animals were eating an unusual mushroom, one that grew from the body of dead caterpillars. An intrepid tribesman decided to experiment for himself. He ate a *Cordyceps sinensis,* found the results satisfactory, and recommended it to his companions. Soon all the tribespeople were eating the mushroom. Their stamina improved and they suffered less from respiratory and other illnesses. The tribespeople shared the newly discovered mushroom with monks of their acquaintance, who shared it with other monks, and soon the reputation of *Cordyceps sinensis* spread throughout China. Eventually, the miracle mushroom landed in the hands of the Emperor's physicians, who prescribed it to the Emperor. Thereafter, by decree, *Cordyceps* could be taken only in the Emperor's palace. All who obtained the mushroom were required by law to turn it over to officers of the Emperor.

Ancient texts describe a couple of unusual ways to take *Cordyceps.* One recipe called for the mushroom to be soaked in yellow wine to make a tonic for the relief of pain in the groin and knees. Another described preparing *Cordyceps* in the belly of a male duck. People suffering from cancer or fatigue were instructed to stuff eight and a half grams of a whole *Cordyceps* mushroom, with the caterpillar casing still attached, into the belly of a newly killed duck, and boil the duck over a slow fire. After the duck had been boiled, the patient was to remove the cordyceps and eat the duck meat for eight to ten days until healthy. Eating duck this way is supposed to have been the medicinal equivalent of taking thirty grams of ginseng (ginseng is probably the most prized medicine in the Chinese pharmacopoeia).

Here is a traditional Chinese recipe for preparing *Cordyceps*:

Cordyceps Duck

12 grams *Cordyceps sinensis*
1 duck (750 grams)
White wine (a dash)
Scallions (2 tablespoons)
Chicken stock (1 quart)
Ginger (1 tablespoon)

Soak the *Cordyceps* in lukewarm water until it is soft. Meanwhile, boil the duck thoroughly. Place the duck in a new pot along with the cooking wine, scallions, soup stock, and ginger. Add salt. Seal the pot tightly and steam for three hours. When done, remove the ginger and scallions. Add pepper.

Foraging for *Cordyceps* with Malcolm Clark

When we brought up the *Cordyceps* mushroom's reputation as a "yak-rodisiac" to mycologist Malcolm Clark, he suggested that *Cordyceps* is likely not what makes the yaks rut in springtime. Clark said that probably the yak seeks out *Cordyceps sinensis* for the same reason that the female pig seeks out the truffle. The animal knows instinctively that eating the mushroom promotes good heath.

"*Cordyceps* is the yaks' medicine," he said, "and they know it. No one has proven that it is an aphrodisiac. The yaks know that *Cordyceps* has some kind of medicinal effect on their bodies."

In 1996, Clark was privileged to accompany members of the Mykot tribe as they foraged for *Cordyceps sinensis* in the Himalayas. Clark is a partner in Gourmet Mushrooms, Inc., a Sebastopol, California, company that supplies specialty mushrooms for the culinary and health food markets. A native of Scotland, he studied biology at university. Since coming to California in 1977, Clark has become one of the premier suppliers of culinary mushrooms to the restaurant trade.

"The Mykots have no written language," Clark explained, his voice betraying a slight Scottish lilt. "Their history is recorded by song. They immigrated to Nepal long, long ago from Tibet. Like all Nepalese, they keep yaks, but the yaks are herded, not fenced. At a certain time of the year, when the snowmelt comes, the yaks start heading up the hill and there is no way of holding these yaks back. They climb to fourteen, fifteen, sixteen thousand feet to find the *Cordyceps*. Most of the mushrooms we collected on our trip were collected between twelve and fourteen thousand feet. We had to go over high passes and that was tough. Three steps forward, rest, three more steps, rest."

To prevent altitude sickness, Clark's companions urged him to eat the *Cordyceps* mushroom. "I ate fresh *Cordyceps* right out of the soil, because the Mykot told me it would help with altitude sickness. I never got sick," Clark said.

"As the Mykot travel with the yaks, they look for a certain kind of primrose that blooms at high elevation. If the primrose isn't blooming, the *Cordyceps* is not going to be out, and you may as well turn around and go back because without the primrose there is no *Cordyceps*."

Sure enough, when they came to where the primrose was growing, the yaks ate the grasses, the yaks ate the primrose flowers, the yaks ate the *Cordyceps*, and the yaks began mating.

Among mycologists, there is a debate as to whether the *Cordyceps* fungus grows outside the caterpillar or is ingested and grows from the inside. Clark believes that the caterpillars actually ingest the *Cordyceps* spores. "When dissecting the caterpillars, I found color variation in the tissue always in more or less the same place. That leads me to believe that the spore is ingested. It gets down through the esophagus and into the gut of the caterpillar, where it germinates. You can actually see the spot of inoculation where germination takes place. I always find one spot on the larvae which is softer and a different color, so what I'm proposing is that it's ingested and it germinates from the inside, where it grows almost like a tuber. It splits the caterpillar's head and grows out through there. When the ground starts to warm in the spring, the *Cordyceps* breaks through the ground and the mushroom appears."

Clark's idea is that *Cordyceps*—the fungus itself—is actually composed of three different organisms. "The theory is that the three work together symbiotically. We may be talking about a yeast or another fungus. It's not been determined what these organisms are. I'm hoping there'll be a breakthrough as far as separating the active parties in the next couple of years."

The Mykots make a yogurt out of *Cordyceps*. They milk the yaks, skim the fat from the milk, and soak dried *Cordyceps* in the milk overnight. In the morning, the milk turns to yogurt.

"As we know, yogurt is made from lactobacillus, or bacteria; it coagulates the proteins. But lactobacillus is not present in the yogurt that the Mykot make from *Cordyceps*. Some kind of enzymatic action keeps it from happening. We haven't found out why; perhaps *Cordyceps* yogurt presents an opportunity for a new health food product."

"Most of the collection spots we went to are hundreds of years old," Clark said about his *Cordyceps*-gathering expedition. "I accompanied the Mykots on the condition that I would not reveal where they harvest the *Cordyceps*. These were secret areas. I'm sure they wanted to blindfold me one or two times. It was a wonderful experience."

Cordyceps and Traditional Chinese Medicine

For many centuries, *Cordyceps* has been the herb of choice in China for treating kidney and lung ailments. In traditional Chinese medicine, *Cordyceps* is said to go directly to the kidneys and lungs, the kidneys being the "root of life," and the lungs being the "Qi of the entire body." (Chapter One of this book outlines the central ideas of traditional Chinese medicine.) *Cordyceps* is considered a potent herb in the pharmacopoeia of traditional Chinese medicine.

Lungs are thought to rule the Qi, which is associated with the element of air. Qi flows without obstruction through the lungs when the lungs are in a healthy state, but if the Qi current is impaired or obstructed by a throat or lung ailment, a defect in nothing less than the body's life force can result. What's more, because the throat is looked upon as door to the lungs and the home of the vocal cords, nose and throat disorders are treated by way of the lungs. For that reason, *Cordyceps,* which goes directly to the lungs and kidneys, is sometimes prescribed for nose and throat disorders.

The kidneys are judged as especially important in traditional Chinese medicine because they store *Jing,* the prime organic material that is neither yin nor yang and is the source of regeneration in the body. All the organs of the body are completely dependent on the kidneys for their life activity. The natural weakening of *Jing* over time brings about old age. Erectile dysfunction, sterility, and reproductive problems are brought about when the kidneys do not store *Jing* properly. Kidneys control the bones and produce bone marrow. Even normal breathing requires the assistance of the kidneys. Because the kidneys are so central to Chinese notions of good health and bodily function, *Cordyceps,* the herb that goes to the kidneys, is prescribed for many ailments.

Cordyceps in the West

The West's first encounter with *Cordyceps* occurred in the early eighteenth century when Father Perennin Jean Baptiste du Halde, a Jesuit priest, brought back specimens from China to his native France. During his stay in the Emperor's court, Father Perennin took a lively interest in *Cordyceps.* Very likely, his curiosity about the mushroom came about when he was prescribed it during a grave illness. According to his diary, Father Perennin, very ill with a fever, had the good fortune to come upon an emissary to the Great Palace in Beijing who happened to be on an errand to deliver *Cordyceps.* The man offered Father Perennin the *Cordyceps* and he soon recovered.

In his diary, Father Perennin wrote that *Cordyceps* can "strengthen and renovate the powers of the system that have been reduced either by overexertion or long sickness." He noted how rare *Cordyceps* was in China, how it had to be imported from the mountainous kingdoms of Tibet, and how it was worth four times its weight in silver.

Upon his return to France, Father Perennin published an account of his experiences with *Cordyceps* and the beneficial effect it had on his health. His report caused a small sensation in the French scientific community. In his report, a mushroom had been shown to have an association with an insect for the first time. The discovery opened the door to the idea of using microorganisms to control crop pests.

The first indication of the origin of *Cordyceps* didn't occur in the West until 1843, when the Reverend Dr. M. J. Berkeley, writing in the *New York Journal of Medicine*, solved the riddle of the mysterious insect-plant. Berkeley noted that the root of *Cordyceps* is indeed a caterpillar, but that the caterpillar had been taken over almost entirely by the mushroom's mycelium.

Cordyceps probably made its debut in the United States in the mid-1800s when Chinese immigrants began arriving to build the railroads. Records show that Chinese physicians were prescribing *Cordyceps* in Oregon and Idaho. The first to market the mushroom were the Lloyd brothers of Cincinnati, Ohio. The brothers, the leading producers of herbal medicines in the United States at the turn of the twentieth century, solicited information about *Cordyceps* from a botanist in China named N. Gist Gee and used the information in their promotional literature. Gee explained that the mushroom was carried down from the mountains of Tibet by tribespeople who collected it at twelve to fifteen thousand feet. He wrote that Chinese doctors recognized it as "good for protecting the lungs, enriching the kidneys, stopping the flowing or spitting of blood, decomposing phlegm produced from persistent coughing, and curing consumption."

Cordyceps Cs-4

Beginning in the 1960s, Chinese mycologists undertook extensive research on *Cordyceps* with an eye toward isolating the most potent strain. Because *Cordyceps* is rare and difficult to collect in the wild, the mycologists' goal was locate a superior strain to supply the ever-increasing worldwide demand for the mushroom. In 1972, researchers at the Institute of Materia Medica of the Chinese Academy of Medical Sciences developed, tested, and finally decided on a strain that they called *Cordyceps Cs-4*, or simply *Cs-4*. The strain was chosen because it is closest to wild *Cordyceps* in the similarity of its chemical components and in its beneficial qualities as an herbal medicine.

Cordyceps Cs-4 was selected from among two hundred other strains of the mushroom. It was isolated from natural *Cordyceps* found in Qing-hai Province, a remote area that was renowned for its *Cordyceps* for many centuries. *Cs-4* meets rigorous standards for safety, grows rapidly using many different cultivation techniques, and resists contamination. More than two thousand patients with various medical disorders were involved in clinical trials of *Cs-4* in China. It became the first traditional Chinese medicine to be approved under China's new and stringent medical standards. In 1987, China's Ministry of Public Health approved *Cs-4*—or *jinshuibao,* as it is known in China—for use by the general population.

Look for *Cordyceps Cs-4* when you are shopping for *Cordyceps sinensis* products in the health food store. By doing so, you can be sure that you are getting a potent and safe variety of *Cordyceps* in the formula you buy.

Recent Studies of *Cordyceps*

Cordyceps has proven useful against a variety of diseases. The mushroom, which grows under trying conditions at high altitude, seems to impart some of its vitality and strength to the people who take it. Following are recent studies that have been done on the *Cordyceps sinensis* mushroom.

Cordyceps and Cholesterol

As nearly everyone knows, a diet high in saturated fats can cause high cholesterol levels. Because most people have trouble managing their diets, it is difficult for most people to lower their cholesterol. Often, prescription drugs are needed, but patients can also take health supplements such as *Cordyceps* to bring down the level of cholesterol in their blood. *Cordyceps,* combined with rigorous exercise and a well-balanced diet, especially one rich in fish, can be a big help in managing atherosclerosis.

In general, *cholesterol* refers to the fatty, waxlike material that is produced by the liver, whose job is to perform vital functions such as hormone production and cell renewal. The liver produces most of the cholesterol that the body needs, but some of it is also obtained from animal products. Sometimes you hear the terms "good cholesterol" and "bad cholesterol." *High-density lipoprotein cholesterol,* or HDL, is the good cholesterol. It appears that HDL cholesterol transports fats, or lipids, through the body so that they can't collect. Bad cholesterol, known as *low-density lipoprotein cholesterol,* or LDL, tends to deposit fats on the blood vessel walls, where it can cause atherosclerosis. What's more, when LDL is deposited in the liver, it can cause fatty liver tissue.

Atherosclerosis is caused when fatty cholesterol deposits form on the artery walls. The artery walls scar and may grow thick with lesions and abrasions called *fibrous plaques.* Eventually, the plaques grow so large that they block the flow of blood to vital areas of the body. What's more, immune cells and muscle cells that normally serve to keep the arteries healthy find their way to the plaques instead. Cell debris also gets stuck in the plaques. Eventually large clumps known as *thrombi* appear on the cells walls. When they break away and enter the bloodstream, a hole is left in the artery wall that can result in hemorrhaging and sudden death.

It appears that *Cordyceps* helps prevent atherosclerosis by decreasing the number of platelets that can get caught in the plaques. *Cordyceps* does this by reducing the viscosity of the blood. In one study, coronary heart disease patients were given three grams of *Cordyceps* a day for three months. They showed a significant drop in blood viscosity and a twenty-one percent drop in total cholesterol.

Clinical studies have shown that *Cordyceps* can increase the amount of good HDL cholesterol and reduce the amount of bad LDL cholesterol in subjects of all ages. The largest study conducted on *Cordyceps* and cholesterol took place in China. In the study 273 patients received one gram of *Cordyceps* three times a day. Cholesterol levels among the subjects dropped by seveneen percent on average when the eight-week trial was complete.

Chinese physicians have also used *Cordyceps* to treat *hyperlipidemia,* a disease caused by high levels of fat in the blood. How *Cordyceps* acts to treat this disease is not well understood, but it does help people who suffer from high cholesterol. In two placebo-controlled trials conducted in China, patients aged sixty to eighty-four were given *Cordyceps* to see how the mushroom would affect age-related oxidation of fats in the bloodstream. After subjects took the *Cordyceps,* doctors discovered that the subjects' red blood cells had significantly higher levels of an enzyme called *superoxide dismutase,* or SOD, one of the body's natural antioxidants. SOD levels in the subjects rose to a level found in seventeen- to twenty-year-olds.

The good news for people who suffer from high cholesterol is that researchers have discovered that lowering cholesterol levels restores the inner lining of the arteries and allows them to relax from the stiffened, plaque-infested state. Apart from administering cholesterol-lowering agents such as niacin and cholestipol, exercise can have a significant effect on cholesterol levels. In one study, twenty-six men with high cholesterol were asked to ride a stationary exercise bike three times a week. The men, all older than forty-six years of age, rode the bike for different amounts of time according to their levels of fitness. Twenty-four weeks into the exercise program, the subjects' cholesterol levels had dropped by nine percent.

Cordyceps and Diabetes

Diabetes, an autoimmune disorder, is associated with abnormally high blood sugar levels. Autoimmune disorders occur when the immune system incorrectly distinguishes between what does and what doesn't belong in the body. In the case of diabetes, T cells incorrectly attack the cells of the pancreas that produce insulin, with the result that the body cannot regulate the buildup of sugar in the blood. Cordyceps, by calming and quieting the cells of the immune system, may be able to help against autoimmune disorders such as diabetes. However, research into the treatment of diabetes with *Cordyceps* is fairly new and much work remains to be done.

The first experiments in treating diabetes with *Cordyceps* were undertaken in Japan and China in the 1990s when scientists reported significant hypoglycemic, or sugar-lowering, effects from the mushroom. In one clinical study involving forty-two diabetics, twenty received an herbal formula that included mycelium powder from *Cordyceps*, and the remaining twenty-two received the herbal formula only (the researchers did not say which ingredients were in the formula). The trial ran for thirty days. At the end of that time, the formula-only group showed symptomatic improvements in 54.5 percent of cases; in the *Cordyceps*-and-formula group, improvement was seen in ninety-five percent of cases (only one diabetic did not improve). Researchers ran tests for *proteinuria*, the urinary excretion of proteins, at the end of the treatment period. Proteinuria is a general indicator of disease advancement. Its presence in diabetics can mean that the patient develops secondary complications such as kidney disease, liver disease, and heart disease. In the study, researchers found a 16.7 percent increase in the rate of proteinuria in the formula-only group; only half the diabetics in the *Cordyceps*-and-formula group showed evidence of proteinuria.

Cordyceps appears to lower blood sugar levels, which is good news for patients who suffer from diabetes. However, patients who tend to be hypoglycemic should use the mushroom only after careful consultation with a physician. If you have a tendency to fatigue or anorexia, your blood sugar levels may already be too low. Taking *Cordyceps* may intensify this problem and cause unwanted health complications.

Cordyceps and Cardiac Arrhythmia

Cardiac arrhythmia is a disturbed or abnormal heartbeat. The most common type of arrhythmia, atrial fibrillation, affects more than two million Americans. Fifteen to twenty percent of strokes in the United States are caused by atrial fibrillation. The disease has many causes, including acute intoxication, hyperthyroidism, and rheumatic valvular disease. Medications such as antipsychotic drugs and antidepressants can increase the risk of arrhythmias, as can high doses of nicotine, caffeine, and other stimulants. Some studies show that blood anticoagulants such as aspirin and warfarin may prevent stroke in arrhythmia patients.

In 1994, a clinical trial was undertaken at Guangzhou Medical College in China to see whether *Cordyceps* can be used to treat ventricular arrhythmia. For the most part, Chinese doctors do not use double-blind placebo-controlled trials, the preferred method of scientific study in the West. In this kind of trial, one group is given a placebo and another group is given a genuine dose of the substance being tested, and results in the two groups are compared. But in the Guangzhou Medical College study, sixty-four subjects were assigned at random to two groups; the test group was given 1,500 milligrams of *Cordyceps* every day for two weeks, and the other group received a placebo. More than eighty percent of patients who were given *Cordyceps* improved, whereas only ten percent of patients in the placebo group recovered. The remaining patients showed no change.

In another study at Guangzhou Medical College, patients with arrhythmia took 1,500 milligrams of *Cordyceps* per day for two weeks. An amazing 74.5 percent of subjects showed improvement. Doctors undertook another trial on thirty-eight elderly patients to see how *Cordyceps* would affect them. This time, subjects took 3,000 milligrams of *Cordyceps* per day for three months. Of twenty-four patients suffering from a type of arrhythmia called supraventricular arrhythmia, twenty showed improvement, with their electrocardiograms, or EKGs, demonstrating a partial or complete recovery. The medical status of three patients who suffered from a complete blockage of the right branch of the cardiac nervous system also improved. From this study, researchers concluded that the benefits of *Cordyceps* increase over time. The longer a patient takes it, the more his or her condition will improve.

Researchers at the Department of Internal Medicine at Hunan Medical University in China undertook a clinical study in 1990 on thirty-seven arrhythmia patients to see if wild *Cordyceps* could help them. Nineteen patients were cured, six in the first week and thirteen in two to three weeks, while the remaining eleven patients showed no improvement.

Cordyceps and Hepatitis B

About 350 million people worldwide are believed to suffer from hepatitis B. According to the World Health Organization, the number will soon reach 400 million. An estimated one million people die each year from the disease.

Hepatitis B is usually contracted by infected blood and sexual contact. It is the number one cause of liver cancer, chronic hepatitis, and cirrhosis of the liver. A vaccine for hepatitis B is available, but it is too costly for most people who live in Africa, Southeast Asia, and China, where the disease is most prevalent. In those parts of the world, an estimated eight percent of the population will die from hepatitis B; over fifty percent of the population will contract the disease in their lifetime. In the United States, approximately 1.25 million people suffer from chronic hepatitis B.

Even when the immune system is able to destroy infected cells and stop the hepatitis B virus from replicating, certain immune cells called *cytotoxic T lymphocytes* may act against the virus without destroying infected cells in the liver. In this case, something more is needed to prevent infected cells from becoming cancerous, especially in chronically infected people. The immunostimulant alpha-interferon is the main treatment for hepatitis B, but it is costly and effective only in about thirty percent of cases.

There is evidence that *Cordyceps* can treat some cases of hepatitis B. In one study, eighty-three subjects aged two to fifteen who carried the hepatitis B virus but showed no symptoms were given *Cordyceps* for three months. A complete conversion of antibodies to the virus was found in thirty-three of the test subjects, which indicates that the infection had been completely resolved and the virus was no longer contagious. Meanwhile, researchers reported that the number of antibodies positive for the virus had decreased in forty-seven percent of the subjects. Because the subjects were so young and their immune systems were not as developed, the drop in the number of positive antibodies indicates that the benefits of *Cordyceps* may well have been more significant than the study showed. Researchers believe that the greater a person's immune response, the less likely he or she is to become a chronic carrier of hepatitis B. Only three to five percent of the adults exposed to hepatitis B become chronic carriers, because their immune systems are developed. Ninety-five percent of infected newborns, by contrast, become chronic carriers. In children under six, about thirty percent become chronic carriers. The drop of forty-seven percent indicated by the study is indeed significant.

In 1990, a study was undertaken in which thirty-two hepatitis B sufferers were given 3,750 milligrams of *Cordyceps* a day for thirty days. Positive antibodies to the virus changed to negative in twenty-one patients. In twenty-three patients, tests showed that liver function had improved.

Cordyceps and Cirrhosis of the Liver

Cirrhosis of the liver is a degenerative disease that is caused by scar tissue in the liver. People who drink alcohol to excess or suffer from hepatitis are subject to the disease. Sufferers are a hundred times more likely to develop liver cancer. About thirty percent of sufferers eventually succumb to liver cancer or complications as a result of chronic active hepatitis B.

Cordyceps has proved to be beneficial to patients suffering from post-hepatitis cirrhosis. This disease sometimes results when the liver does not heal correctly after a bout of hepatitis.

In 1986, an extract of cultured mycelium was tested in twenty-two patients with post-hepatitis cirrhosis. Patients took six to nine grams of *Cordyceps* every day for three months, and by the end of the study, their symptoms had improved dramatically. Cirrhotic cells had disappeared in fifteen patients, and had decreased significantly in another six patients.

In a more recent study, Japanese and Chinese researchers found that mice developed a high-energy state in their livers, without signs of toxicity, after consuming large quantities of *Cordyceps* mycelium. The researchers concluded that one of the main effects of taking *Cordyceps* on a repeated basis might be a higher metabolic state of the liver. One drug prescribed to treat cirrhosis, called malotilate, helps the liver regenerate by activating the cells of its energy factories. This in turn boosts concentrations of an essential enzyme called ATP. The fact that *Cordyceps* causes increases in ATP levels may be one way it helps repair the liver.

Cordyceps and Fatigue

Chinese athletes have begun to use *Cordyceps* as general health supplement to increase vitality and energy and as a post-exercise recovery food. In traditional Chinese medicine, doctors have long used the mushroom to treat cases of excessive tiredness. *Cordyceps* seems to increase patients' stamina. For this reason, physicians have recently been looking into whether *Cordyceps* can aid patients who suffer from chronic fatigue syndrome.

Although the disease is a recognized disorder, chronic fatigue syndrome is difficult to diagnose accurately. Its strong psychological component has made it a controversial subject in Western medicine. No single test or biological aspect has yet determined the presence of chronic fatigue syndrome, and the biochemical and biological signs of the disease are sure to be a subject of debate for years to come. Complicating the problem of diagnosis, fatigue can be caused by any number of diseases, including low blood pressure, AIDS, tuberculosis, depression, and/or hepatitis.

By definition, a person is diagnosed with chronic fatigue syndrome if he or she exhibits these symptoms:

- The patient has shown signs of the disease for more than six months.
- The patient is not tired by reason of overexertion.
- The patient can get no relief by resting.
- The patient suffers from at least four of the following ailments: headache, muscle pain, unrefreshing sleep, memory impairment, inability to concentrate, post-exertion malaise, sore throat, multijoint pain, or tenderness of the auxiliary lymph nodes or cervical nodes.

More research needs to be done to determine the effectiveness of *Cordyceps* in alleviating fatigue. In the meantime, however, people suffering from fatigue who have tried *Cordyceps* have reported some encouraging results. How does *Cordyceps* help people who suffer from chronic fatigue? Scientists report that chronic fatigue syndrome sufferers have an unusual form of adrenal insufficiency and, strangely, high levels of male hormones. Because *Cordyceps* improves the function of the adrenal cortex, it may help people who suffer from chronic fatigue syndrome. The mushroom also strengthens the resiliency and integrity of the HPA (hypothalamic-pituitary-adrenal) axis, the neuroendocrine system that responds to stressful events by producing chemical messengers that bring feelings of despair. It appears that *Cordyceps* calms the HPA axis and thus the nervous system.

In any case, *Cordyceps* does appear to boost the stamina of people who are not suffering from chronic fatigue. At the annual meeting of the American College of Sports Medicine in 1999, Dr. Christopher Cooper, Professor of Medicine and Physiology at the UCLA School of Medicine, presented a study that showed how *Cordyceps sinensis* increases exercise performance. In the study, thirty healthy elderly patients underwent a double-blind, placebo-controlled trial in which they were tested on a cycle ergometer. Subjects who took *Cordyceps* increased their oxygen intake from 1.88 to 2.00 liters per minute; those who took the placebo showed no increase in oxygen intake. Dr. Cooper concluded, "These findings support the belief held in China that *Cordyceps sinensis* has potential for improving exercise capacity and resistance to fatigue. The results complement other studies which have shown increased cellular energy levels through the use of *Cordyceps*."

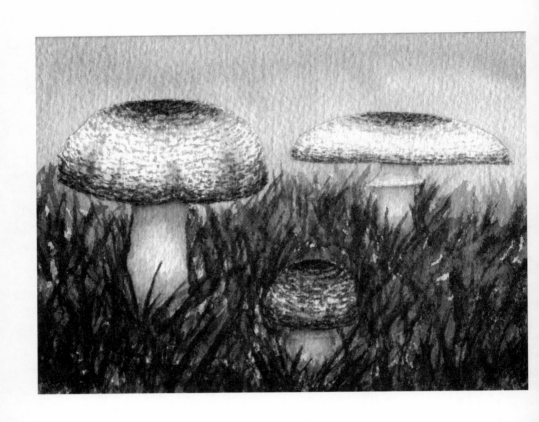

CHAPTER FIVE

Agaricus Blazei

Beta Glucan All-Star

ONE OF THE MOST exciting medicinal mushrooms is a relative new-comer, *Agaricus blazei*. Many scientists believe that the beta glucan in this mushroom is more potent than that of other mushrooms. Forty years ago, the medicinal properties of the mushroom were known only to a few thousand villagers in Brazil, but since the world discovered the mush-room, its reputation has spread far and wide. *Agaricus blazei* has shown real promise as an immunomodulator and a defense against tumors.

Discovery of *Agaricus Blazei*

Agaricus blazei does not have as colorful a past as some of the other mushrooms described in this book. Instead of the exotic East, the ori-gins of *Agaricus blazei* can be traced to a small mountain town in Brazil called Piedade located some 120 miles (200 km) southeast of São Paulo. For centuries, the inhabitants of the town and its environs have savored a mushroom that they call *Cogumelo de Deus* ("the mushroom of God"), *Cogumelo do Sol* ("the sun mushroom"), *Cogumelo Princesa* ("the princess mushroom"), or *Cogumelo da Vida* ("the mushroom of life").

In 1965, two events transpired to bring the rare mushroom to the attention of the world. In the summer of that year, a Brazilian farmer of Japanese descent named Takahisa Furumoto was roaming the mountains beside Piedade when he noticed an unfamiliar but tasty mushroom. The mushroom appeared to be of the *Agaricus* family. Furumoto sent spores of the mushroom to Inosuke Iwade of the Iwade Research Institute of Mycology in Japan. To learn more about the mushroom, Iwade, a scholar in the field of mushroom cultivation, attempted to grow the mushroom in his laboratory, an attempt that would take nearly a decade.

Meanwhile, back in Piedade, a group of scientists led by Dr. W. J. Cinden of Pennsylvania State University had begun their own investigation into the unknown *Agaricus* mushroom. Cinden and his colleagues had come to Piedade to find out why the inhabitants of the town had low rates of geriatric disease and a reputation for longevity. He concluded that the people of Piedade enjoy long life because they eat an unusual mushroom of the *Agaricus* family as part of their diet. Dr. Cinden published his findings in *Science* magazine and presented his conclusions at several conferences. Word about the unusual mushroom from Brazil began to spread.

After Inosuke Iwade at last managed to cultivate samples of the *Agaricus* mushroom in his laboratory in Japan, he noticed that this *Agaricus* was longer and thicker than others in the *Agaricus* family. The gills took longer than usual to turn black. The mushroom emitted a strong aromatic odor and the root was sweet and delicious. Did he have a new species on his hands? Iwade submitted a sample of the mushroom to a Belgian taxonomist named Heinemann, who deemed the mushroom a new species of *Agaricus*. He named it *Agaricus blazei* Murrill because, as it turned out, the mushroom had already been documented and described by the noted American mycologist W. A. Murrill. According to the story, Murrill found the mushroom on a lawn in Gainesville, Florida. (As a staff member of the New York Botanical Garden in 1904, Murrill identified the infamous Chestnut blight, *Endothia parasitica*, the fungus that all but destroyed the American chestnut tree, "queen of the Eastern forest," in the eastern United States. From the 1930s until his death in 1957, Murrill discovered over 650 species of fungi in Florida.)

Agaricus blazei grows in the southeastern United States, although not as prolifically as in South America. In Japan, the commercial name of the mushroom is *Himematsutake;* its common name is *Kawariharatake*. It is also known by these names: Murrill's agaricus, Royal sun agaricus, and, less frequently, songrong and almond portobello.

Problems in Cultivating *Agaricus Blazei*

Agaricus mushrooms are quite common throughout the world. The "button mushroom" (*Agaricus bisporus*) found in American supermarkets is an example of an *Agaricus* mushroom. There are about thirty species of *Agaricus*. The mushrooms range in color from off-white to light brown. The caps emerge as round "buttons" from the soil and grow in size from one to twelve inches across, depending on the species. At first the gills are off-white, but within three days they turn pink, purple, and then black. Chances are, if you see a mushroom growing on a lawn or pasture, it is an *Agaricus* mushroom.

Agaricus blazei, however, does not grow as wantonly as most *Agaricus* mushrooms. Where other species of mushroom prefer shade and dampness, *Agaricus blazei* favors the humid, hot-house environment of its native Brazil. The mushroom grows only in the hot summer months. It may die if temperatures drop too low. In the Piedade region, temperatures range from 95 degrees (35C) during the day to 72 degrees (22.2C) at night, and the land receives a good dousing by tropical rain in the afternoon or early evening. According to a story, one reason that *Agaricus blazei* thrives in the region has to do with the number of wild horses found there. Horse manure, the story goes, contributes to the fertility and unique composition of the soil.

Attempts to cultivate the mushroom with biotechnological assistance did not begin producing stable yields until the 1990s. *Agaricus blazei*'s tropical native environment is very difficult to replicate. The mushroom is now being cultivated in Japan, Korea, the United States, Denmark, Holland, and Brazil. Sugarcane bagasse was found to be the best culture bed material for growing the mushroom. A few years ago, when the demand for *Agaricus blazei* skyrocketed and its price rose accordingly, the mushroom all but disappeared from the Piedade region of Brazil, according to some reports. (Another story had it that horse manure never stayed on the ground long in Piedade—it was needed by farmers for the cultivation of *Agaricus blazei*.)

The Beta Glucan in *Agaricus Blazei*

As Chapter Two of this book explains, beta glucan is a kind of polysaccharide chain molecule that is found in medicinal mushrooms. Beta glucan is known to help make the immune system more alert and balanced.

Although no one knows for certain how beta glucan does its work, it is believed that beta glucan fools the immune system into thinking it is being attacked by a bacterium. The immune system, accordingly, marshals its defenses, and the result is a stronger immune system.

Some scientists believe that *Agaricus blazei* contains the highest level of beta glucan of any mushroom. Many studies seem to show that the beta glucan in *Agaricus blazei* is especially advantageous against tumor cells. Due to its low molecular weight, beta glucan from *Agaricus blazei* can be absorbed into the body more easily than beta glucan from other mushrooms. This is believed to make it more effective.

Recent Studies of *Agaricus Blazei*

Clinical interest in *Agaricus blazei* began in earnest when a study showing antitumor activity by the mushroom was presented at the general convention of the Japanese Cancer Association in 1980. In the study, *Agaricus blazei* was reported to have higher levels of beta glucan than the maitake (described in Chapter Six of this book), shiitake (Chapter Ten), or reishi mushroom (Chapter Three).

In 1995, Dr. Mamdooh Ghoneum of UCLA Medical Center, speaking at the Ninth World Immunology Congress, declared that the *Agaricus blazei* mushroom increases the total number of all immune cells within the body and also makes individual natural killer cells more powerful. This was a startling announcement in many ways, because it was the first time that a prominent American researcher had sung the praises of *Agaricus blazei*. Also in 1995, at the Seventh General Meeting of the Technical Discussion Group for Fungi held in Nara, Japan, Dr. Takashi Mizuno, who has studied *Agaricus blazei* for many years, commented on a beta glucan he isolated in the mushroom, "The glucan-protein complex was the first case of an antitumor compound found in an edible mushroom."

Agaricus blazei has indeed generated a lot of interest in the scientific community. Following are recent studies concerning the medicinal qualities of the mushroom.

Agaricus Blazei and Cancer

Cancer is a complex immune-associated disease that can affect any organ or system of the body. It is caused by uncontrolled cell growth resulting from a genetic defect or cellular damage due to radiation or toxins in the environment. Although many advances have been made in the field of cancer research, there is still much to be done. Unfortunately, treatments such as radiation and chemotherapy can be as debilitating to the patients as the cancer itself. Research indicates that traditional therapy used in combination with alternative therapies may help cancer patients.

Scientists at Kobe Pharmaceutical University in Japan decided to test the effects of *Agaricus blazei* on cancer. They injected a water-soluble fraction from *Agaricus blazei* into one group of cancerous mice and a saline solution into another group. Results of the experiment showed an increase in lymphocyte T cells, the immune system cells that are involved in protecting humans against cancer, in the *Agaricus blazei* group. As Chapter Two of this book explains, lymphocytes are carried in the lymph, the fluid that circulates in the lymphatic system.

The scientists concluded that beta glucan from *Agaricus blazei* may be an effective preventative against cancer. In other words, if your family is predisposed to getting breast cancer or prostate cancer, taking *Agaricus blazei,* especially early in life, may be a good idea, as it may keep you from developing the cancer.

Agaricus Blazei and Tumors

Some herbal extracts, including those from mushrooms, are known to attack tumors without doing any damage to normal tissue. In 1999, a group of scientists from Japan extracted substances from *Agaricus blazei* in order to monitor their effect on tumors in laboratory mice. The scientists injected the tumor with the *Agaricus blazei* substances and noticed a marked inhibition in the tumor in the right flank where they made the injection and in the left flank as well. One of the components of the *Agaricus blazei* extract was a polysaccharide complex with a low molecular weight called Alpha-1, 4-Glucan-Beta, 6-Glucan. The scientists reported that this polysaccharide had the strongest antitumor effect. It was able to selectively kill tumor cells without affecting normal cells.

Interestingly, the experiment also showed the possible activation of granulocytes. *Granulocytes* contain *granules* with potent chemicals that kill micro-organisms and play a role in controlling acute inflammatory reactions. The scientists speculated that both flanks of the tumor were inhibited because the granulocytes were able to migrate to the left flank, the side of the tumor where the injection was not made. It seems that the *Agaricus blazei* polysaccharide examined in the study not only inhibits tumors from growing, but it also stimulates the migration of the white blood cells that scavenge and kill malignant cells.

The same group of Japanese scientists conducted a similar experiment with *Agaricus blazei* extracts. This time, the noninjected side of the tumor also regressed, but the scientists noted that it regressed due to the activation of natural killer cells. What's more, the extract induced apoptosis in the malignant cells. In effect, *apoptosis* refers to cells committing suicide. Again, in this experiment, the scientists observed that the *Agaricus blazei* extract killed tumor cells, but not healthy ones. Apoptosis was seen only in the malignant cells.

Another *Agaricus Blazei* Cancer Study

To immobilize or neutralize a malignant cell is not enough. The body needs to rid itself of the cell by making it burst and killing it. One way that the body destroys cells is by way of *complement*, a series of proteins that are produced in the liver. The activation of the complement cascade causes holes to be punched in the membrane of the targeted cell and its inside to ooze out. The most active component of complement is called C3. Complement also attracts and stimulates macrophages to eat the malignant cells. As Chapter Two explains, macrophages are the giant white blood cells that eat and destroy malignant cells.

Recently, scientists at Mie University School of Medicine in Japan conducted experiments to gauge the effect of *Agaricus blazei* on complement proteins made in the liver. Specifically, they wanted to examine the activity of the C3 complement. The scientists implanted sarcoma tumors in mice and fed the mice a polysaccharide that they cultured from the mycelia of *Agaricus blazei*. The polysaccharide succeeded in activating macrophages in the mice and activating C3 protein. From this, the scientists concluded that *Agaricus blazei* could well be an aid in fighting the spread of malignant cancer cells in the body.

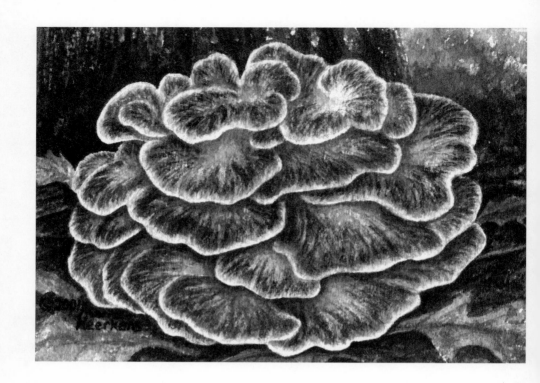

CHAPTER SIX

Maitake

The Cancer Slayer

MAITAKE (MY-TAH-KAY) MEANS "dancing mushroom" in Japanese (*mai* means "dance"; *take* means "mushroom"). How the mushroom got its name depends on which story you choose. In one account, the mushroom got its name because people danced with joy upon finding maitake mushrooms in the forest. They may well have danced with joy during Japan's feudal era, when local lords paid tribute to the shogun by presenting him with maitake mushrooms, among other gifts. To obtain the maitake mushrooms, the local lords are supposed to have offered anyone who found one the mushroom's weight in silver—a cause for dancing indeed. Another story says that the dancing mushroom got its name because the overlapping fruit-bodies give the appearance of a cloud of dancing butterflies.

In the English-speaking world, maitake is known as Hen of the Woods. The mushroom, growing as it does in clusters, is said to resemble the fluffed tail feathers of a brooding hen. Less frequently, the mushroom is called Sheep's Head. It is sometimes called the "king of mushrooms" on account of its size. The mushroom's Latin name is *Grifola frondosa*. *Grifola* is the name of a fungus found in Italy. Some scholars believe that the fungus got its name from the griffin (or griffon), the mythological beast with the head and wings of an eagle and the hind legs and tail of a lion. *Frondosa* means "leaflike." The overlapping caps of maitake mushrooms growing in the wild give the appearance of leaves.

Maitake in the Wild

The chief characteristic of the maitake mushroom is the fact that it grows in clusters. The caps, which are typically four to five inches across, overlap one another to form a sort of clump. The stems, meanwhile, fuse together. Maitake grows at the base of oak trees, beeches, and other dead or dying hardwoods. According to folklore, the mushroom prefers to grow where lightning has scarred the wood of a tree. A typical maitake cluster is the size of a volleyball. Clusters can be twenty inches in diameter and weigh as much as eighty pounds.

The mushroom prefers temperate northern forests. It is indigenous to northeast Japan, Europe, Asia, and the eastern side of the North American continent. Connoisseurs favor maitake mushrooms from Japan for their flavor.

Commercial techniques for the cultivation of maitake mushrooms were not perfected until the late 1970s. Before then, the only way to harvest maitake was to pick it in the wild. Foragers in Japan were said to be very covetous of the secret places where maitake grew. To mark their forest turf and keep others away, foragers cut hatch marks into trees. Known locations of maitake were called "treasure islands." Where to find these "treasure islands" was a carefully guarded secret. Many a forager kept the secret his entire life and revealed it only in his will so that his eldest son could find his way to the treasure.

Recent Studies of Maitake

Maitake is a delicious culinary mushroom, but the Japanese also value it for its medicinal properties. Traditionally, maitake was used in Japan as a tonic to boost the immune system and increase vitality. The mushroom was supposed to prevent cancer and high blood pressure. For that reason, researchers turned their attention to maitake's effect on those diseases when they first began experimenting with maitake three decades ago.

In recent years, the maitake mushroom has become a popular subject of study. In a search of Medline, the online service of the National Library of Medicine, we found more studies pertaining to maitake than to any other mushroom covered in this book. Following is a look at recent studies of the maitake mushroom that we think are important.

Maitake and Diabetes

Diabetes is caused by abnormally high levels of glucose, or sugar, in the blood. The disease is an example of an autoimmune disorder in which the immune system does not function properly and works contrary to itself. Diabetes is brought about when immune-system cells mistakenly attack the cells in the pancreas responsible for producing insulin, the hormone that is in charge of converting sugar into energy. The result is a sugar buildup in the body, as the body is unable to burn off excess blood sugar. An estimated 16 million Americans have diabetes and the disease contributes to nearly 200,000 deaths annually. Symptoms include excessive thirst, frequent urination, fatigue, a tingling sensation in the hands and feet, and unexplained weight loss.

To find out if maitake has any effect on diabetes, researchers in Japan fed powder from the fruit-body of the mushroom to diabetic mice. The mice received one gram of powder a day (very little, considering that a mouse eats one third its weight daily). The researchers discovered a decrease in blood sugar in the mice. What they found most interesting about their experiment, however, was an increase in insulin production on the part of the mice. It appears that maitake can help diabetes sufferers in two different ways. Maitake increases the production of insulin and controls glucose levels as well—in mice at least. We look forward to experiments with maitake on human diabetes sufferers.

A warning: People who have diabetes will be glad to know that most mushrooms, maitake included, appear to lower blood sugar levels. However, if you are hypoglycemic—if you have *low* blood sugar levels— you should take maitake only after consulting a physician. Taking maitake may bring your blood sugar levels even lower and cause health complications. Dizziness, fainting, sweating, headaches, and malaise are symptoms of hypoglycemia.

Maitake and Cholesterol

People who have a diet that is high in saturated fats run the risk of getting high cholesterol levels in their blood. High cholesterol can lead to hyperlipidemia, atherosclerosis, and other health problems. Cholesterol is a fatty, waxlike material that is produced by the liver. It is essential for cell renewal, hormone production, and other important bodily functions. There are two kinds of cholesterol. High-density lipoprotein cholesterol (HDL), the good cholesterol, carries lipids—that is, fat—through the blood and keeps lipids from collecting. Low-density lipoprotein cholesterol (LDL), the bad cholesterol, deposits lipids in the liver and on the walls of blood vessels where it can accumulate and cause harm.

Maitake mushrooms may have an inhibiting effect on the production of lipids, and therefore have the ability to lower cholesterol levels. Scientists at Kobe Pharmaceutical University in Japan ran experiments on two groups of mice with hyperlipidemia. Both groups were fed a high-cholesterol diet, but one group's diet was supplemented with maitake powder. The maitake-fed mice had fewer lipids in their livers *and* their blood. An interesting sidelight of the experiment was the effect of the maitake on good cholesterol in the maitake-fed mice. Usually, levels of HDL cholesterol decrease under the effect of a high-cholesterol diet. In the case of the maitake-fed mice, however, HDL cholesterol levels remained the same.

Maitake and Prostate Cancer

The problem with any malignancy, including prostate cancer, is that the malignant cells do not want to die. They want to live forever and they want to proliferate. This can be very dangerous.

Recently, scientists from the Department of Urology at New York Medical College in Valhalla, New York, conducted experiments to study the effect of maitake on prostate cancer cells. The scientists isolated and grew hormone-resistant prostate cancer cells. The cells were then treated in vitro with a highly purified beta glucan extract from maitake called Grifon-D. After twenty-four hours, the scientists examined the prostate cancer cells and discovered that almost all of them had died.

The scientists also wanted to know how the Grifon-D extract from maitake worked in combination with vitamin C. Their experiments produced an interesting result: Vitamin C may make maitake more effective. By including vitamin C in the dose, the scientists were able to get the same results—death of the majority of prostate cancer cells—with one-eighth the amount of Grifon-D. Vitamin C appears to enhance the antioxidant effect of maitake (as Chapter Two explains, antioxidants help reverse the damage that free radicals do to body tissue). The scientists concluded that beta glucan from maitake may have use as an alternative therapy for prostate cancer.

Maitake and Bladder Cancer

Researchers at Gunma University in Japan conducted an experiment to determine the inhibiting effect of different mushrooms on bladder cancer. For the experiment, laboratory mice were fed a carcinogen called BBN every day for eight weeks. BBN is known to cause cancer of the bladder. The rats were divided into four groups. One group was given no mushroom supplement, one was given shiitake mushrooms, one maitake mushrooms, and one oyster mushrooms (*Pleurotus ostreatus*).

After eight weeks, the scientists examined the rats to see which had developed bladder cancer. In the group that received no mushroom supplement, 100 percent had contracted cancer. In the maitake group, 46.7 percent (seven of fifteen mice) developed cancer; in the shiitake group, 52.9 percent (nine of seventeen mice) developed cancer; and in the oyster group, 65 percent (thirteen of twenty mice) developed cancer. In terms of protection against cancer of the bladder, maitake works better than shiitake and oyster mushrooms.

The experiment also yielded interesting results concerning macrophages, the powerful immune-system cells that attack foreign materials. Normally, macrophages move to their prey in much the same way that a dog comes running when it smells food. Macrophages are attracted to cells that appear to be foreign. Carcinogens such as BBN, however, suppress macrophages' ability to find foreign cells quickly. Carcinogens numb the activity of macrophages. This experiment, however, revealed that mushrooms actually protect macrophages from being numbed. Among mice who had received mushroom supplements in their diet, macrophages were still very hungry and active despite being exposed to the carcinogen BBN.

The three mushrooms in the experiment had a similar effect on lymphocytes, the white blood cells that circulate in the lymph nodes and flush viruses and bacteria from the body. Lymphocyte activity in the group of mice that did not receive a mushroom supplement was impaired, but the lymphocytes in the other mice maintained a normal level of activity.

Maitake and Obesity

Obviously, maintaining the right body weight is important for your health. According to the United States Centers for Disease Control, obesity—defined as being thirty percent or more above ideal body weight—increased from twelve percent of the population in 1991 to 17.9 percent in 1998. Why are many people obese? One reason has to do with genetics. Some genes are associated with obesity. Environmental factors also come into play. In the United States, time spent in front of the television can genuinely be considered a cause of obesity. Television broadcasts messages that encourage people to eat fast food, foods of dubious nutritional value, and foods loaded with "empty" calories. Television watchers are sedentary. Between eating the fast food that the television encourages them to eat and the idle time they spend in front of the television, television viewers are prone to gain weight.

Recently, scientists at Mukogawa Women's University in Nishihomiya, Japan undertook an *in vitro* experiment to see what effect maitake had on certain kinds of cells. For the experiment, the scientists focused on the $C3H10T1/2B2C1$ cell. This cell is normal in most aspects, but it has the potential to balloon and turn into an *adipocyte,* a kind of fat cell. You could say that $C3H10T1/2B2C1$ cells have the potential to become obese. For that reason, observing this kind of cell is useful for determining how substances effect weight loss and weight gain. The results of the experiment showed that maitake inhibits the conversion of normal $C3H10T1/2B2C1$ cells into adipocytes. It appears that maitake lowers the risk of becoming obese to a certain extent. The mushroom may also be useful to people who want to lose weight or maintain their weight.

In a study conducted at the Koseikai Clinic in Tokyo, thirty-two overweight subjects were given 10 grams of maitake powder for two months to see if they would lose weight. Without changing their diets, all subjects lost weight, with the average loss being twelve pounds.

Maitake and the Liver

As "Medicinal Mushrooms and Prebiotics" in Chapter Two explains, the average person carries three to four pounds of bacteria in his or her gastrointestinal tract. Some of these bacteria are actually good for the body. They help prevent constipation and diarrhea, for example. Bad bacteria, however, are also present in the gastrointestinal tract. Certain types of bad bacteria produce a substance called *D-galactosamine.* This substance is associated with inflammation and liver toxicity. Physicians can determine how much damage D-galactosamine has caused by testing for certain enzymes in the blood. If these enzymes are present in large numbers, the liver has been damaged.

In an experiment to see whether medicinal mushrooms can suppress the effects of D-galactosamine on the liver, scientists from Shizuoka University in Japan used D-galactosamine to damage the livers of laboratory rats. Then they fed the rats various medicinal mushrooms for two weeks to find out which mushrooms worked best at suppressing D-galactosamine. They discovered that maitake works best. What's more, the effects of maitake were dose-dependent. In other words, the larger the dose of maitake given to the rats, the better the effect it had on suppressing D-galactosamine.

This experiment seems to indicate that maitake can help protect the liver against the effects of bad nutrition. If you eat fast foods or foods that are low in fiber, taking maitake may be able to improve the health of your gastrointestinal tract and protect your liver from damage caused by D-galactosamine.

Maitake and Its Effect on the Immune System

Researchers have known for some time that 1-3 beta glucan aids the immune system and that 1-3 beta glucan from different mushrooms aids the immune system in different ways. Maitake, for example, stimulates macrophages to produce more cytokines. As we explained in Chapter Two, macrophages are powerful cells of the immune system that engulf and destroy foreign organisms and substances. Cytokines are the messengers of the immune system. They alert the immune system to the presence of an invader. In some cases, they also kill foreign cells.

Recently, scientists from the Tokyo University of Pharmacy and Life Science conducted in vitro experiments to observe the behavior of a certain kind of cytokine called tumor necrosis factor alpha, or TNF alpha. This toxinlike substance is especially adept at killing malignant tumor cells. The scientists wanted to see what effect maitake had on the production of TNF alpha. They already understood that macrophages must first eat beta glucan before they release TNF alpha and other cytokines. What the scientists discovered is that macrophages release TNF alpha only after they have eaten a certain kind of high-molecular-weight beta glucan. A study along the same lines conducted at Tokyo College of Pharmacy concluded that small-molecular-weight beta glucan from the maitake mushroom serves to prime the cells of the immune system and get them ready for an attack. Yet another study from Tokyo College of Pharmacy looked at interleukin 6, or IL-6, another cytokine known for its effectiveness against tumor cells. This study noted that maitake stimulated the production of IL-6.

These important studies confirmed that not all beta glucans activate the immune system in the same way; some beta glucans are specialized. We look forward to experiments that examine the effect of specific types of beta glucan on specific parts of the immune system.

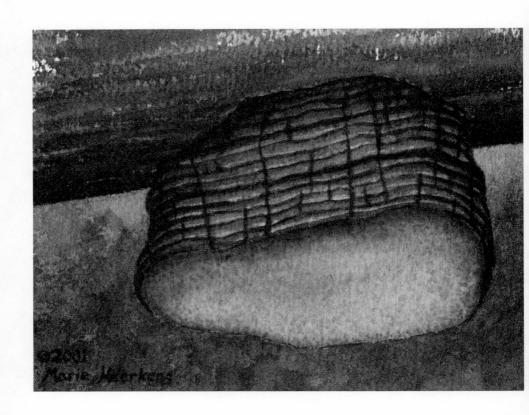

©2001
Marie Heerkens

CHAPTER SEVEN

Phellinus Linteus

New Superstar on the Block

UNTIL QUITE RECENTLY, *Phellinus linteus* was almost unknown outside the Korean peninsula. The mushroom is a relative newcomer and a rising superstar. For several hundred years, Korean physicians prescribed *Phellinus linteus* as a treatment for cancer, stomach ailments, and arthritis. In traditional Korean medicine, the mushroom is known to ease pain caused by inflammation. One medical text recommends it as a means of treating a red nose brought about by the immoderate drinking of alcohol. News of the mushroom's medicinal properties began reaching the outside world in the 1970s, when studies concerning *Phellinus linteus* were published in the Japanese and Chinese scientific press. In the past decade, manufacturers of Korean health-food products have marketed the mushroom aggressively, so convinced are they of its medicinal benefits. Teports about the mushroom's value as treatment for arthritis have been circulating among herbalists in the United States and Europe for some time.

An interesting sidelight of *Phellinus linteus* is the mushroom's part in bringing together scientific and commercial interests from North and South Korea. The governments of those nations, who are not known for cooperating with one another, have permitted teams of scientists from both nations to conduct joint research. South Korea's Unification Ministry has permitted some business concerns from the south to import *Phellinus linteus* mushrooms from the north. Perhaps the healing properties of the mushroom touch the political as well as the biological.

A Quick Look at *Phellinus Linteus*

Phellinus linteus is a thick, hard, woody, hoof-shaped mushroom with a bitter taste. It has a pale brown to light yellow cap. The stem is thick and varies in color from dark brown to black. The mushroom favors dead or dying mulberry trees and is found in Korea and adjacent parts of China. Traditionally, the mushroom is boiled in water and is taken as a tea. Koreans sometimes soak it in wine or whisky before drinking it. *Phellinus linteus* is used as an ingredient in skin creams because it is believed to rejuvenate the skin. The etymology of the mushroom's Latin name is as follows: *Phellinus* means "cork"; *linteus* means "linen cloth."

Recent Studies of *Phellinus Linteus*

As we noted at the start of this chapter, studies in *Phellinus linteus* are few and far between because the mushroom is a relative newcomer. Still, one or two interesting studies have been presented in recent years.

Phellinus Linteus, Tumors, and Metastasis

As Chapter Two of this book explains, mushroom polysaccharides help awaken the immune system and keep it alert. To be specific, they help what is called the cell-mediated part of the immune system—the macrophages, lymphocytes, natural killer cells, and so on. They also help the humoral part of the immune system, the part that is mediated by the antibodies that plasma cells secrete.

The general activity of mushroom polysaccharides on the cell-mediated and humoral parts of the immune system is well understood. Recently, scientists in South Korea decided to go a step further and see if *Phellinus linteus* could work alongside Adriamycin, a popular chemotherapy drug, to inhibit tumors. They were especially interested in *metastasis,* the movement of tumor growth from one location in the body to another by way of blood circulation or the lymphatic system. The scientists wanted to see if *Phellinus linteus* in combination with Adriamycin could inhibit metastasis. For the experiment, they implanted melanoma tumors in laboratory mice. They fed one group of mice *Phellinus linteus* and Adriamycin, one group *Phellinus linteus* alone, and one group Adriamycin alone. Then the scientists looked at the growth of tumors in the mice, their survival rate, and the frequency of metastases in their lungs. Here are some of the findings of their study:

· Mice who took *Phellinus linteus* alone had a higher survival rate. In this group, tumor growth was inhibited and the frequency of metastases was reduced.
· In mice who took Adriamycin alone, tumor growth was significantly inhibited, but metastasis was only slightly inhibited.
· The combination of *Phellinus linteus* and Adriamycin was effective in inhibiting tumor growth, but not in inhibiting metastasis.
· *Phellinus linteus* did not kill cancer cells directly.

The scientists concluded that *Phellinus linteus* might be of use in conjunction with chemotherapy drugs such as Adriamycin. Although *Phellinus linteus* doesn't work directly to kill tumors, it does help the immune system work better. Therefore, the mushroom might be useful as an adjunct to chemotherapy and other anticancer treatments.

Phellinus Linteus Compared with Other Beta Glucans

One of the most interesting questions facing scientists who investigate the medicinal qualities of mushrooms is how the beta glucans from the different mushrooms enhance the immune system. As we have written repeatedly in this book, different mushrooms affect the immune system differently.

In 1999, scientists in Korea conducted an in vivo and in vitro experiment to compare the activity of beta glucan from *Phellinus linteus* with beta glucan from *Basidiomycete* fungi. They conducted the tests both on laboratory mice and in culture. The scientists found the following in regard to *Phellinus linteus:*

· Increased activity by T lymphocytes and cytotoxic T cells, the white blood cells that destroy viruses and cells that have been mutated by cancer

- Increased activity by natural killer cells and macrophages
- Stimulation of the production of B cells, which in turn produce more antibodies to combat disease

Phellinus linteus appears to exhibit a wider range of immunostimulation than other polysaccharides. It stimulates both the cell-mediated and the humoral parts of the immune system. The mushroom is indeed a potent one.

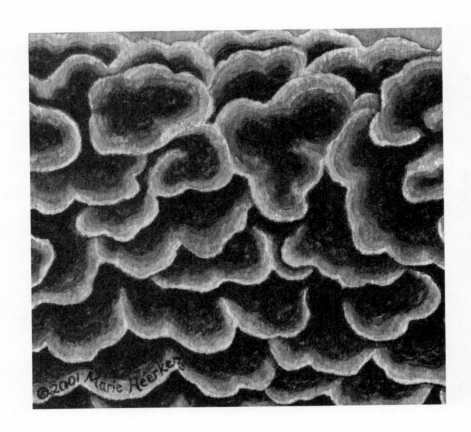
©2001 Marie Heerkens

CHAPTER EIGHT

Trametes Versicolor

The Mother of Krestin

Trametes versicolor HAS THE distinction of being the mushroom from which one of the world's leading anticancer drugs is derived. The drug is called Krestin. Although Krestin has not been approved for use by the United States' Food and Drug Administration (FDA), it was the best-selling anticancer drug in Japan for much of the 1980s, with sales topping $500 million annually. Krestin was the first mushroom-derived anticancer drug to be approved by the Japanese government's Health and Welfare Ministry, the equivalent of the United States' FDA. All healthcare plans in Japan cover members' purchases of Krestin.

    Trametes versicolor came to the attention of the pharmaceutical industry in 1965 when a chemical engineer working for Kureha Chemical Industry Company Ltd. in Japan observed his neighbor attempting to cure himself of gastric cancer with a folk remedy. The neighbor was in the late stages of cancer and had been rejected for treatment by hospitals and clinics. For several months, he took the folk remedy, a mushroom, and then, having been cured, he went back to work. The folk remedy was *Trametes versicolor.*

    The engineer from Kureha Chemical convinced his colleagues to examine the mushroom. The best strain of *Trametes versicolor* was found and cultivated. Soon PSK, an extract from the mushroom, was born. PSK is the chief ingredient in Krestin. PSK stands for *Polysaccharide-K*, *K* being the first letter of Kureha Chemical, the company that developed PSK and Krestin. As Chapter Two explains, a polysaccharide is a chain molecule constructed from sugar units. One-three beta glucan, the type of polysaccharide found in medicinal mushrooms, is especially beneficial to the immune system.

The success of Krestin inspired Chinese researchers to look into and develop an extract from *Trametes versicolor* of their own. This extract is called PSP. PSP stands for *Polysaccharide-Peptide*. In biochemistry, a *peptide* is a compound of low molecular weight that figures in the creation of proteins. PSK and PSP are derived from different strains of *Trametes versicolor*. What's more, the extraction methods and fermentation processes of each substance are different. Clinical experimentation with PSP did not begin until the early 1990s, whereas clinical studies of PSK have been conducted since 1978.

Introducing *Trametes Versicolor*

Trametes versicolor is found in temperate forests throughout the world and in all fifty states of the United States. It is lovely and is occasionally included in floral displays. In the English-speaking world, the mushroom is known as the Turkey Tail because its fan shape resembles the tail of a standing turkey. It is striped with dark-to-light brown bands that alternate with bands of orange, blue, white, and tan. It prefers to grow on dead logs and has been known to feed on most kinds of trees.

In Latin, the etymology of *Trametes versicolor* is as follows: *Trametes* means "one who is thin"; *versicolor* means "variously colored." In some literature, the mushroom is called *Coriolus versicolor* and, rarely these days, *Polyporus versicolor*, but taxonomists now agree that the mushroom should properly be *Trametes*, not *Coriolus* or *Polyporus*. In China, the mushroom is called *yun zhi*, or "cloud mushroom." In Japan it is called *Kawaratake*, which means "beside the river mushroom."

The Japanese have long used *Trametes versicolor* as a folk remedy for cancer. In traditional Chinese medicine, *Trametes versicolor* is used to treat lung infections, excess phlegm, and hepatitis. The ancient Taoists revered the mushroom because it grows on pine trees. Because pines are evergreens, Taoist priests assumed that the mushroom had the staying power of the pine tree, which never loses its foliage. Taoists believed that *Trametes versicolor* collects yang energy from the roots of the pine tree, and they prescribed it for patients whose yang energy was deficient.

A Look at PSK and Krestin

At the fourteenth annual International Chemotherapy Symposium in 1991, no less than sixty-eight papers about PSK were presented, about a fifth of all papers. In those heady days, it seemed as though PSK and Krestin might unlock the secret to preventing cancer and helping cancer patients recover.

The drug is almost always prescribed to cancer patients who have had a tumor removed and are undergoing chemotherapy or radiotherapy. It is often prescribed for colon, lung, stomach, and esophagus cancer and has no side effects. Chemotherapy and radiotherapy damage the bone marrow and thereby interfere with the production of blood cells, including white blood cells, which play an important role in the immune system. Following are three recent studies that demonstrate the effectiveness of PSK on cancer patients' immune systems:

- In a ten-year study of 185 lung cancer patients who were undergoing radiotherapy, Japanese doctors administered Krestin to roughly half the patients (the others got a placebo). The idea was to see whether Krestin could boost the cancer patients' white blood cell activity and thereby strengthen their immune systems. After ten years, thirty-nine percent of patients who had Stage I or II lung cancer and took Krestin survived; only sixteen percent survived in the non-Krestin group. Of Stage III cancer patients, twenty-two percent survived in the Krestin group; only five percent of the patients who did not take Krestin survived.
- In a randomized, controlled clinical trial of 227 patients with breast cancer, doctors prescribed PSK and chemotherapy for some patients and chemotherapy alone for others. In this ten-year study, 81.1 percent of patients who took PSK and were treated with chemotherapy survived; 64.5 percent of patients who had chemotherapy alone survived.
- In a five-year study of 262 stomach cancer patients who had gastrectomies (a removal of part of the stomach), some patients received PSK along with their chemotherapy treatment and

some did not. Of the patients who received PSK, seventy-three percent were still living after five years. The survival rate of the other group was sixty percent. The study concluded that PSK along with chemotherapy was "beneficial for preventing recurrence of cancer and in prolonging survival for patients who have undergone curative gastrectomy."

Krestin came under fire beginning in the late 1980s at several medical conventions, where doctors questioned its effectiveness. The substance, it seemed, had been overhyped. The Health and Welfare Ministry in Japan now instructs doctors to use Krestin only as an adjunct to chemotherapy or radiotherapy. The drug by itself is not supposed to be used as a treatment for cancer.

PSK can raise survival rates in cancer patients and prolong their lives. Moreover, the substance is nontoxic. Because the risk to patients of taking PSK appears minimal and the rewards are many, PSK is likely to be an aid in fighting cancer for years to come.

A Look at PSP

Like PSK, PSP is prescribed to cancer patients to help improve their immune systems before and after surgical treatment, chemotherapy, and radiotherapy. China's Ministry of Public Health approved PSP as a national class I medical material in 1992. In 1999, PSP was added to the list of medicines whose cost could be reimbursed by government medical insurance and the labor medical insurance programs. What's more, the National Cancer Research Center in the United States has declared PSP a fungous anticancerous substance. The PSP that has been researched here is derived from a special strain of *Trametes versicolor* called COV-1. Here are a couple of recent studies concerning PSP:

- Scientists at the University of Shanghai studied 650 cancer patients who were undergoing chemotherapy or radiotherapy to see if PSP could ameliorate the side effects of their treatment. Using twenty criteria for assessing adverse reactions to anticancer drugs—weakness, night sweats, and others—the scientists determined that the PSP group had markedly fewer side effects than the control group.
- In a placebo-controlled study, researchers at the Shanghai Institute of Chinese Medicine administered PSP to one group under-

going chemotherapy or radiotherapy for cancer and a placebo to another group. Then they observed both groups for evidence of anorexia, vomiting, dryness of throat, and other side effects, as well as increased weight, higher natural killer cell counts, and other signs of improvement. What the researchers called "the overall effective rate"—the rate at which patients' health improved—was significantly higher in the PSP group at 85.8 percent than the control group at 41.9 percent.

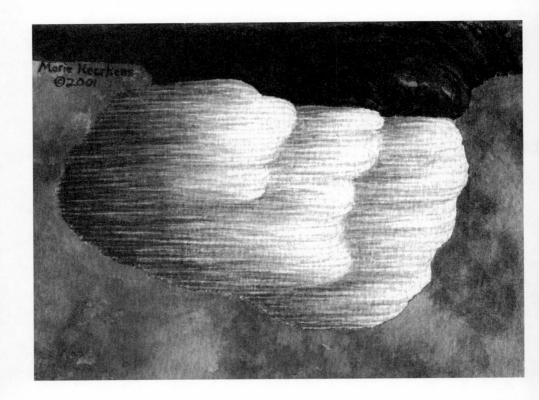

CHAPTER NINE

Hericium Erinaceus

A Cure for Alzheimer's Disease?

Hericium erinaceus IS FOUND throughout the Northern Hemisphere in Europe, East Asia, and North America. The mushroom's exotic, otherworldly appearance has inspired admirers to give it a host of unusual names: Lion's Mane, Monkey's Mushroom, Monkey's Head, Bear's Head, Hog's Head Fungus, White Beard, Satyr's Bear, Old Man's Beard, Bearded Hedgehog, Hedgehog Mushroom, Pom Pom (because it resembles the ornamental pom-pom ball on the end of a stocking cap), and Pom Pom Blanc (because *Hericium erinaceus* is white to off-white in color). In Japan, the mushroom is known chiefly as *Yamabushitake. Yamabushi*, literally "those who sleep in the mountains," are hermit monks of the *shugendo* sect of ascetic Buddhism. *Hericium erinaceus* is supposed to resemble the *suzukake*, an ornamental garment that these monks wear. *Take*, the other half of *Yamabushitake*, means "mushroom" in Japanese. In China, the mushroom goes by the name *shishigashira*, which means "lion's head," and *Houtou*, which means "baby monkey." In some literature, *Hericium erinaceus* is mistakenly called *Hericium erinaceum*.

The mushroom is two to eight inches across. Its white, iciclelike tendrils hang from a rubbery base. A sharp knife is often needed to remove the mushroom from the hardwood from which it grows. The mushroom favors dead or dying broadleaf trees such as oak, walnut, and beech. Recently, *Hericium erinaceus* was blamed in northern California for an outbreak of heart rot in live oak tress.

In traditional Chinese medicine, *Hericium erinaceus* is prescribed for stomach disorders, ulcers, and gastrointestinal ailments. A powder extract from the mushroom called *Houtou* is sold in China. In North America, Native Americans used *Hericium erinaceus* as a styptic. The mushroom was commonly found in Native Americans' medicine bags. Dried powder from the mushroom was applied to cuts and scratches to stop them from bleeding.

Hericium erinaceus is a culinary as well as a medicinal mushroom. To some, it gives the hint of seafood, crab or lobster. The mushroom has a rubbery texture similar to squid. The commercial cultivation of *Hericium erinaceus* began quite recently. Until two decades ago, the mushroom was considered a rare find in the forest, but now its name can be found on the menus of gourmet restaurants.

Travels with *Hericium Erinaceus*

As we mentioned, Chinese pharmacies carry pills and powders that are made from *Hericium erinaceus*. Very likely the people who take these powders don't realize that they are taking powder cultivated with techniques developed in Sonoma County, California. How the *Hericium erinaceus* got from Sonoma County to China makes for an interesting story and it also illustrates how mycologists share information about medicinal mushrooms.

In 1980, a fellow mycologist informed Malcolm Clark that he had seen an unusual fruiting of *Hericium erinaceus* on a tree in Glen Ellen, a small town in Sonoma County some fifty miles north of San Francisco. Clark, co-owner and founder of Gourmet Mushrooms, Inc., had long been cultivating mushrooms for the gourmet market. He was told that the *Hericium erinaceus* specimen grew on a bay tree that had fallen over a winter creek. Clark, seizing the opportunity to study *Hericium erinaceus* first-hand, took his sleeping bag and some instruments from his lab in Sonoma County to the site in Glen Ellen and camped there for three days.

"I just watched the thing for a while," he said. "I lived with it. It was important for me to be with the mushroom."

Clark took observations regarding sun exposure, light, and humidity. He measured the mushroom. After the three days were over, he harvested the mushroom and took it back to his lab. There, Clark cultured the *Hericium erinaceus* specimen.

"I was able to make up a substrate and fruit the mushroom according to what I had been able to observe," he recounted. "Then it was a case of improving it to find out how much better I could make it grow and under what control conditions."

Clark's chief interest in *Hericium erinaceus* at this time was developing the mushroom for the culinary market. He took it to Ernie's Restaurant in San Francisco, where then chef Jacky Robert took one look at the mushroom and exclaimed, "Ah, Pom Pom Blanc." Clark trademarked the name. Pom Pom Blancs are now available in many gourmet restaurants.

Recent Studies of *Hericium Erinaceus*

Western science opened the book on *Hericium erinaceus* a few short years ago. Although the mushroom has been part of the diet in Japan and China for many centuries and its medicinal properties as a styptic are well known, scientists have hardly begun to study it. However, the mushroom has turned a few heads for its unusual medicinal properties. In a recent article in the *International Journal of Medicinal Mushrooms*, Dr. Takashi Mizuno of Shizouka University in Japan noted the following about *Hericium erinaceus:*

- Owing to their effect on the immune system, polysaccharides from the fruit-body of the mushroom may help against stomach, esophageal, and skin cancer. These polysaccharides modulate the immune system so that it responds more effectively and helps people who have cancer to control the disease and manage the side effects of chemotherapy.
- Preliminary studies show that low-molecular-weight pharmaceutical constituents such as phenols (hercenon A and B) and fatty acids (Y-A-2) from *Hericium erinaceus* may have chemotherapeutic effects on cancer. These molecules seem to operate directly against cancer cells.

What was especially intriguing about Takashi Mizuno's article was its implications for the treatment of Alzheimer's disease. Some four million Americans, including former President Ronald Reagan, suffer from this affliction, the most common form of irreversible dementia. Symptoms of Alzheimer's disease include confusion, memory loss, disorientation, and the inability to speak or reason. Scientists believe that the disease is caused in the brain by plaque buildup around nerve cells and by tangled up nerve fibers called *neurofibrillary tangles.* Alzheimer's disease has no known cure, and it is always fatal.

Dr. Mizuno reported that compounds in *Hericium erinaceus* may encourage the production of a protein called *nerve growth factor* (NGF). This protein is required in the brain for developing and maintaining important sensory neurons. To put it simply, *Hericium erinaceus* may regenerate nerve tissue in the brain. For this reason, compounds in the mushroom may be useful in the treatment and prevention of Alzheimer's disease. We look forward to more studies in this area.

Hericium Erinaceus and the Immune System

Recently, scientists at Zhejiang College of Traditional Chinese Medicine in Hangzhou, China, undertook an experiment to find out whether *Hericium erinaceus* can activate T and B lymphocytes in the immune system. These white blood cells circulate in the lymph and blood and flush viruses and bacteria from the body. The scientists were interested in knowing how *Hericium erinaceus* affected the lymphocytes and what would happen if the mushroom were used in conjunction with other substances known to stimulate lymphocyte production.

The scientists isolated T and B lymphocytes from the blood of laboratory mice. They placed these lymphocytes in test tubes and spiked the test tubes with various combinations of a lectin called Con-A, polysaccharides from *Hericium erinaceus,* and lipopolysaccharide (LPS), another white-blood-cell stimulant. The scientists observed the following:

- *Hericium erinaceus* polysaccharides and Con-A together made the T lymphocytes proliferate at three times the rate they proliferated when Con-A alone was placed in the test tube. *Hericium erinaceus* alone, without Con-A, had no effect on lymphocytes.
- *Hericium erinaceus* polysaccharides and LPS together made lymphocytes proliferate at two to three times the rate they proliferate with LPS alone. Once again, *Hericium erinaceus* polysaccharides alone had no effect on lymphocyte production.

From this experiment, it appears that *Hericium erinaceus* can play a role in boosting the immune system when it is used in combination with other substances, namely Con-A and lipopolysaccharide (LPS).

Hericium Erinaceus and Sarcoma Tumors

To test the effectiveness of *Hericium erinaceus* on tumors, scientists at the Kyoritsu Pharmaceutical & Industrial Co. in Japan transplanted sarcoma tumors into laboratory mice and fed the mice different doses of dried mushroom powder for fourteen days. At the end of the period, they cut out the tumors and weighed them to see if they had grown. The result of their experiment: the tumors either shrank or stopped growing.

The interesting aspect of this experiment, however, had to do with the mushroom's overall effect on the immune system. The scientists concluded that T cells had not shrunk the tumors. *Hericium erinaceus* is not chemotherapeutic. The *Hericium erinaceus* extract worked by stimulating the immune system of the animal, which in turn helped to control and reduce the burden of the sarcoma tumor.

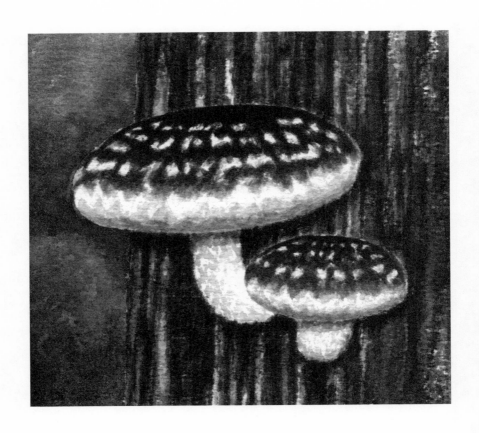

CHAPTER TEN

Shiitake

Lentinan and HIV

HOW THE JAPANESE discovered the health benefits of shiitake makes for an interesting story. In the 1960s, Japanese researchers undertook a series of epidemiological studies to learn everything they could about incidences of disease in their country. In the course of one study, they found two remote mountainous districts where cancer was nearly unheard of. The government sent teams of scientists to these districts to find out why cancer rates were so low there. Was it something about how the people lived? Something in the diet? It so happened that growing shiitake mushrooms was the chief industry in both districts. The inhabitants ate a lot of shiitake, apparently believing that it helped prevent cancer.

The shiitake mushroom is delicious. After the white button mushroom, shiitake is the most popular culinary mushroom in the world. The cultivation of shiitake in the United States is increasing faster than the cultivation of any other culinary mushroom. Shiitake is a gourmet delight. The mushroom's meaty flavor can complement almost any dish and, as it turns out, the mushroom that delights so many with its distinctive flavor is also a medicinal mushroom.

Introducing the Shiitake Mushroom

The mushroom is known throughout most of the world by its Japanese name, shiitake (shee-ee-TAH-kay). The name comes from the Japanese word for a variety of chestnut tree, *shiia*, and the Japanese word for mushroom, *take*. Shiitake is sometimes called the Forest Mushroom and the Black Forest Mushroom. In China, it is known as *Shaingu-gu* (alternate spelling, *Shiang-ku*), which means "fragrant mushroom." Shiitake's Latin name is *Lentinula edodes*, the etymology of which is as follows: *lent* means "supple," *inus* means "resembling," and *edodes* means "edible." About 1980, a debate concerning shiitake's Latin name broke out among taxonomists. Without going into all the details, the mushroom's name was changed from *Lentinus edodes* to *Lentinula edodes*. Prior to 1980, literature concerning the shiitake mushroom refers to the name *Lentinus edodes*.

The shiitake mushroom is native to Japan, China, the Korean peninsula, and other areas of East Asia. The cap is dark brown at first and grows lighter with age. The spores are white and the edges of the gills are serrated. In the wild, shiitake grows on dead or dying hardwood trees—chestnut, beech, oak, Japanese alder, mulberry, and others—during the winter and spring. It prefers forest shade where cold water is nearby. The shiitake industry in Japan, as large as it is, can be credited with preserving much of the nation's forests. Without income from shiitake, many a yeoman farmer would have long ago cut down his trees or sold his land to developers. Shiitake mushrooms are Japan's leading agricultural export. Japan accounts for eighty percent of worldwide shiitake production.

Even by mushroom standards, shiitake is high in nutrition. The mushroom contains all the essential amino acids, as well as eritadenine, a unique amino acid that some physicians believe lowers cholesterol. Shiitake is high in iron, niacin, and B vitamins, especially B1 and B2. In sun-dried form, it contains vitamin D.

Shiitake cultivation in the United States got off to a slow start, thanks in part to the United States Department of Agriculture. For much of the last century, the USDA imposed a complete quarantine on the importation of shiitakes. USDA bureaucrats imposed the quarantine because they mistook *Lentinus edodes* (shiitake's former Latin name; it has since been changed to *Lentinula edodes*) for another mushroom called *Lentinus lepideus*. This mushroom—its common name is Train Wrecker—was known to attack and corrode railroad ties. Train Wrecker was the suspect in several railway mishaps. The USDA realized its mistake and lifted the quarantine against shiitakes in 1972. Today, American growers produce approximately five million pounds of Shiitake mushrooms annually.

Folklore of Shiitake

Historical documents in Japanese archives relate how Chuai, the bellicose fourteenth emperor of Japan, praised the shiitake mushrooms that were given him by members of the barbarian Kumaso tribe, whom he was trying to subdue on the island of Kyushu in the second century. Shiitake is supposed to have been used in the ancient Japanese royal court as an aphrodisiac.

In China, the cultivation of shiitake mushrooms began about a thousand years ago with a woodcutter named Wu San-Kwung in the mountainous areas of Zhejiang Province. To test his axe, Kwung swung it against a fallen log on which shiitake mushrooms grew. Days later, he noticed shiitake mushrooms growing where his axe struck the log. As an experiment, he cut the log in several different places. Once again, shiitake mushrooms grew where his axe landed. In this way, the log method of cultivating mushrooms was born. On one occasion, the story goes, mushrooms failed to grow on a log and Kwung grew frustrated. He attacked the log, beating it vigorously with the blade of his axe. When he returned to the scene of the battering, he discovered to his surprise that the log was covered with mushrooms. Kwung had discovered the "soak and strike" method of mushroom cultivation in which logs are battered in such a way that spores have more openings in which to germinate. This method is still used in some places. Wu San-Kwung's contributions to agriculture are commemorated in a temple in Qingyuan. Festivals in his name are still celebrated throughout Zhejiang Province.

Lentinan and LEM

In traditional Chinese medicine, shiitake is used to treat high cholesterol, atherosclerosis, colds, and flu. The mushroom is also believed to enliven the blood, dispel hunger, and cure the common cold. It is supposed to boost Qi, the primal life-force that animates the body and connects it to the living cosmos. Given the high regard with which shiitake is held, it was only a matter of time before scientists got around to testing its medicinal properties.

In 1969, Tetsuro Ikekawa of Purdue University, working in conjunction with researchers at the National Cancer Center Research Institute in Tokyo, extracted a 1-3 beta glucan from shiitake that he tested on mice that had been infected with tumors. In seventy-two to ninety-two percent of the mice, tumor growth was inhibited. From this study, Lentinan was born (the beta glucan was named for *Lentinula edodes*). Ikekawa and his colleagues conjectured that Lentinan bolstered the immune system by activating macrophages, T lymphocytes, other immune-system cells, and the production of cytokines.

By 1976, scientists had run Lentinan through clinical trials and pharmaceuticalized it. The Japanese government's Health and Welfare Ministry, the equivalent of the United States' Food and Drug Administration (FDA), soon approved the drug and it was put on the market. Almost immediately, Lentinan proved effective in treating many kinds of cancers. However, the drug does not have any direct anticancer activity. When Lentinan is placed in a test tube with cancer cells, it does not affect the cells, but when it is injected into the body, Lentinan triggers the production of T cells and natural killer cells. Lentinan is the third most widely prescribed anticancer drug in the world. Doctors often prescribe it to patients who have undergone chemotherapy as a means of revitalizing the patients' immune systems. Regrettably, Lentinan has not been approved by the United States' Food and Drug Administration. Except under special circumstances, it is not available to Americans.

Shortly after the AIDS epidemic began in the early 1980s, physicians began experimenting with Lentinan as a means of making the immune system less susceptible to HIV, the virus that causes AIDS. Lentinan generated a lot of enthusiasm at the Sixth International Conference on AIDS in 1990, when reports were published showing the drug's ability to increase helper T cells, the cells whose job it is to mark invaders so they can be destroyed by the immune system (HIV destroys helper T cells).

Another substance extracted from shiitake called LEM (*Lentinula edodes* mycelium) is believed to be helpful against hepatitis B. This disease is transmitted by blood transfusions, nonsterilized needles, and sexual contact. Some studies have shown that LEM stimulates the production of antibodies that counteract hepatitis.

Recent Studies of Shiitake

Following are a couple of recent studies that concern shiitake mushrooms. Shiitake is good medicine. Given the popular notion that what tastes good is bad for your health, we wonder if people would find shiitake mushrooms as delicious if they knew how good for their bodies.

Lentinan and AIDS

Aware that a Japanese study showed that cancer patients did not get significant side effects from taking Lentinan, researchers in the United States were curious whether Lentinan could be used to treat AIDS patients. The researchers wanted to know whether Lentinan could strengthen AIDS patients' immune systems and whether the patients would tolerate Lentinan as well as the Japanese cancer patients had. As we mentioned earlier in this chapter, Lentinan is a 1-3 beta glucan that is extracted from the shiitake mushroom.

The study of AIDS patients was conducted jointly in San Francisco and New York. In San Francisco General Hospital, ten patients were intravenously administered either 2, 5, or 10 milligrams of Lentinan or a placebo once a week for eight weeks. At the Community Research Initiative in New York, two groups of twenty patients were intravenously administered either 1 or 5 milligrams of Lentinan twice a week for twelve weeks, and ten patients were administered a placebo. In New York, where the infusion was carried out over a thirty-minute period, no side effects were reported. In San Francisco, where infusion took ten minutes, four patients discontinued therapy because of side effects. Still, most side effects disappeared in twenty-four hours after the medication was discontinued. What's more, dramatic side effects such as anemia, a drop in white blood cells, or inflammation of the pancreas were not observed.

In all patients who took Lentinan, the number of lymphocytes—the white blood cells that circulate in the lymph and help flush viruses and bacteria from the body—went up. However, researchers cautioned that the small number of patients in the study prohibited them from concluding that Lentinan actually increases activity by lymphocytes. Given the small number of side effects observed in the study and the increase in lymphocytes, researchers recommended undertaking a trial in which Lentinan is used in combination with zidovudine (AZT) or didanosine (a protease inhibitor), two drugs specific for HIV.

A subsequent trial in which the researchers treated some patients with Lentinan and didanosine and other patients with didanosine alone showed a marked increase in lymphocytes in the Lentinan-didanosine patients when compared with those who received only didanosine.

These provocative studies suggest that Lentinan can be useful for treating patients with HIV.

Shiitake and Tooth Decay

Dental plaque is a soft, thin, sticky film that forms on the surface of teeth, often near the gum-line. It is made up of millions of bacteria, as well as saliva and other substances, and can cause tooth decay. In case you haven't heard by now, the best way to prevent plaque from forming on teeth is to brush regularly.

To see if shiitake can help prevent tooth decay, researchers from the Nihon University School of Dentistry in Japan conducted a test in which they exposed the *Streptococcus mutans* and *Streptococcus sobrinus* bacteria to shiitake powder. Dentists know these bacteria very well, because they are the primary components of dental plaque. In an in vitro test, researchers observed a decrease in plaque formation in the test tube. In an in vivo test conducted on laboratory rats that had been infected with *Streptococcus mutans,* researchers compared rats who had been fed the shiitake extract with rats who did not get the benefit of shiitake. The researchers discovered significantly fewer cavities in the shiitake group. What's more, the shiitake component of the rats' diet amounted to only 0.25 percent, which indicates that shiitake may be a potent protection against tooth decay.

In another study undertaken at the Nihon University School of Dentistry, researchers found that shiitake was effective against several bacteria, including varieties of *Streptococcus,* that are commonly found in the mouth. Generally speaking, the study found that microbes such as *Candida* that are not found in the mouth were resistant to the mushroom. It appears that as a medical mushroom, shiitake is especially useful to dentists.

CHAPTER ELEVEN

Real Stories and Healing Experiences

DR. FUKUMI MORISHIGE, M.D., Ph.D., is a surgeon who worked at the Linus Pauling Institute in Japan. Here, he tells how reishi helped cure one of his patients of lung cancer:

> In June of 1986, a thirty-nine-year-old female came to me with lung cancer and complications of the chest wall membrane. A number of hospitals had told her that she could not be operated on. She left in a hopeless state. Upon returning home, her husband started to feed her reishi. Six months earlier, she had edema in the chest cavity, secondary to cancer, but now the cancer had completely disappeared. A person who had already made her funeral arrangements and was waiting for death rediscovered there is hope for life—that's incredible. She insisted that [her cure] was the result of her husband giving her reishi.

The following comes from Dr. Banchert Tantivit, M.D. The doctor is a graduate of the University of Oregon Medical School and the author of *Melatonin and I* and *The Lingzhi I Know* (written in Thai).

> This is a case of Mr. Chen, a fifty-five-year-old man from Penang. I interviewed him in front of his two sons in one hotel in Anson Road in Penang in 1997.

Mr. Chen had a sudden heart attack in 1989. Angiographic study reviewed triple coronary artery disease. One tributary was completely blocked. No surgery was advised. He was treated with conventional medicine. After four years, his condition deteriorated. A repeat angiogram showed that the narrowing of the heart arteries was getting worse. Bypass surgery was advised lest he have another heart attack any moment.

The patient was too afraid to have such a major operation. A friend advised him to take *lingzhi* (reishi mushrooms). His friend explained to him, with such serious kind of disease, highly concentrated *lingzhi* had to be taken and in high doses. Finally convinced, he started to take twelve *lingzhi* capsules a day. Then a miracle happened. He began to feel better. The usual fatigue was gone. There was no longer shortness of breath or chest pain. Eleven months after taking *lingzhi,* a third angiogram was taken and showed that there was marked improvement of the coronary artery disease. What was most amazing was that the artery that was completely blocked had opened again.

The following also comes from Dr. Banchert Tantivit:

Here is a case of brain cancer. A thirty-five-year-old, healthy man, my friend's son in Los Angeles, was found to have brain cancer, called *glioblastoma multiforme.* This is one of the most aggressive brain cancers. Most people with this kind of cancer don't survive beyond one year. The patient was treated by a team of doctors from Harvard University. Three therapy techniques were used: cut (surgery), burn (radiotherapy), and poison (chemotherapy). Despite the best efforts by doctors from the famous hospital, the cancer recurred after one year. New experimental chemotherapy was tried. After two sessions, the chemotherapy was discontinued because it was too toxic for the patient. The doctor told the patient's parents that their son would not live long, maybe a matter of weeks.

My friend called me from LA and asked whether there was any herbal medicine that might help his son. I suggested *lingzhi* (reishi). And I told him that the dosage had to be really high. Twenty capsules had to be taken a day instead of the usual three to six. In treating cancers, shock therapy has to be employed; otherwise it won't be effective.

My friend did not have any experience with *lingzhi.* Understandably, he hesitated to accept my advice. After consulting his two other sons (who were doctors) and concluding that there was nothing to lose, he finally decided to follow my advice. Starting in June of 1998, twenty capsules of *jia hor lingzhi* were given daily to the patient. To treat diseases serious and life-threatening such as cancer, a high-quality product has to be used. Now one year and six months have passed, my friend's son is still alive, and he enjoys a reasonably good quality of life. Although he cannot walk without aid because of the damage to the motor nerve of the legs by toxic chemotherapy, and his memory was affected by burn therapy, he is enjoying his life, laughing in front of the television.

The most encouraging news is that the latest brain scan showed that the cancer mass has shrunk somewhat. My friend's son is going to live and enjoy life for many more years.

The following is from Dr. Samuel Yoon, a veterinarian who practices in Western Massachusetts. Dr. Yoon is a highly respected, much-sought-after veterinarian.

Many times chemotherapy or radiation therapy is recommended for animals, but in the case of animals, those treatments are too expensive. Radiation treatment for a dog, for example, can easily run to four or five thousand dollars. Because these treatments are expensive, I started looking for alternatives. I studied acupuncture, and eventually I started looking into herbal treatments.

Six years ago I returned to Seoul, Korea, to attend a course of study. With scholars there, I discussed how to treat cancer with herbal medications. One day I ran across a newspaper ad placed by a pharmaceutical college professor. He claimed that he had extracted an anticancer agent from a mushroom. The mushroom was reishi. When I returned to the United States, I was able to obtain a copy of the reishi study from the professor. I became interested in the healing properties of reishi and other mushrooms. I started using reishi and eventually maitake and shiitake as well.

Ten months ago, I had a bulldog with breast cancer. He was operated on, and chemotherapy was recommended, but it wasn't an option. The dog was too old and we were concerned about its safety. The owners and I agreed to use maitake to cure the dog. Now the dog is as energetic as ever. I couldn't find tumors when I cut open the dog. The dog shows no signs of relapse.

In another case, I treated a sixteen-year-old poodle with a big lump on its hip. I couldn't do a biopsy on the tumor because the dog was so old. It was a do-or-die situation. I prescribed reishi for this poodle. I choose reishi because it probably has more polysaccharides. Do you know how I used it? I injected reishi at the base of the tumor. Nobody had done that before, as far as I know. A week later, the tumor had shrunk by twenty to thirty percent. I made another injection, about 2 or 3 cc. It shrank again by twenty to thirty percent. I made the injection every week for a month. The tumor shrank to the size of a grain of salt. Without the reishi treatment, I would have had to cut out the tumor, and I probably would have lost the dog. The dog lived another three or four years, and the tumor eventually disappeared.

In another case, I had a sixteen-year-old mixed-breed dog with a lump on its ankle. I couldn't operate because of an edema, a tumor pressing against a blood vessel. I injected reishi again. The swelling decreased by forty percent. Of course, I used other medications too, but I doubt if they were solely responsible for reducing the swelling. I injected one more time. The swelling was down another twenty or thirty percent. Now the lump was small enough to be operated on. I cut it out, and it never came back.

I also treated a dog with oral melanoma. It was a large dog, about a hundred pounds. I operated on the dog and put him on maitake, three capsules daily. I didn't find evidence of melanoma for a whole year, but when the owner reduced the prescription to two capsules, the melanoma came back. Unfortunately, the dog died. Maybe the maitake only suppressed the cancer, and the lower dose allowed it to come back.

Andrew H. Miller, age forty-four, is the president of Myco-Herb, Inc. (and a co-author of this book). Miller was interested in the transformational aspects of reishi that the Taoists spoke of so many years ago. His experiences with the mushroom captured for him what it must have been like to the ancient Taoists:

The ancient Chinese medical literature says that reishi can relieve the body of its material weight, prolong life, and transform the person who takes it into a supernatural being.

I felt it was worth a try. I had suffered from chronic lung problems since adolescence. At least twice a year, I would have a bout of bronchitis that was serious enough to warrant a course of antibiotics and bed rest. Once I began taking reishi, there was no looking back. Although I have the occasional cold or flu, I have not had one case of bronchitis since.

Another experience I had with reishi dealt more with the psychic side of my being. I had been told by colleagues that some people experience a "psychic healing crisis" when taking reishi. That one happened to me. Within a few days of taking my course of reishi, I noticed that my dream state was becoming more agitated. I dreamed about people and places and situations that I had long ago forgotten about or buried in my subconscious—unpleasant experiences from my childhood, emotions and anxieties relating to events long forgotten. I would wake up in a cold sweat and lay awake for hours reflecting on these memories, sights, sounds, and even smells that had risen from my subconscious.

The time spent lying awake was, I realize now, the beginning of a profound transformation for me. I had been carrying around a lot of negative psychic burdens, and reishi was expunging them and ridding me of the burden of carrying them around.

While in my waking state, it was as if I was able to detach myself and observe my interactions with other people, as if I were in the audience and on stage at the same time. I was able to see how I interacted with people and subsequently, I was able to change behavior patterns and ways of communicating with other people that I was unhappy with and wanted to change.

Well, I did change. I felt as if the terrain of my mind and body had shifted dramatically. I was not the same person anymore. Reishi calmed my mind, my nerves, and allowed me to concentrate more fully—allowed me, I think, to enjoy life more fully.

Rose Menlowe, age seventy-nine, is the grandmother of Jordan Rubin, founder of Garden of Life, a company that makes revolutionary whole-food nutrition products as well as a multiple-mushroom formula. His RM-10 multiple-mushroom formula is created using the Poten-Zyme process of biofermentation creating enhanced absorption and utilization while also providing beneficial probiotics and enzymes. No other fermentation process like this can be found anywhere. Jordan Rubin formulated RM-10 for his grandmother, Rose Menlowe, after she was diagnosed with metastatic cancer.

Two years ago, I was diagnosed with cancer. The visible tumors were surgically removed and I underwent no further conventional treatment. My grandson formulated a special blend of herbs and probiotics for me to take. He told me that if I took this blend, my immune system and digestion should significantly improve. Whatever it was he gave me, boy did it work! I have been using RM-10 for about eighteen months. I've never felt better in my life. I experience more energy than I ever remember having. I have a general feeling of well-being that I have never experienced. As a side note, I have been constipated all of my adult life. I have always required the use of laxatives, which didn't always help. After a few months of RM-10 I've eliminated the use of my laxatives and have almost perfect elimination. According to my last check-up, I am cancer-free.

CHAPTER TWELVE

Behind the Scenes

THIS CHAPTER TAKES a peek behind the scenes to show you some techniques for cultivating medicinal mushrooms. It also offers advice for buying medicinal mushroom products and explains the virtues of multiple-mushroom formulas. You will meet some of the people who produce the products in this chapter. These pages also offer the strange story of the orgasmic mushroom.

How Medicinal Mushrooms Are Cultivated

For many centuries, foraging for and picking mushrooms in the wild was the only way to obtain them. Sometime in the first millennium, however, cultivators in Japan and China began using the log method to grow mushrooms. With this technique, logs from felled trees are placed next to a stump or log where the fruit-bodies of mushrooms grow. The idea is for spores from the fruit-body to find their way to the felled trees and spawn a new crop. The log method is still practiced in parts of China. People use it to supplement their incomes and produce mushrooms for local markets.

More controlled methods of cultivation begin in the 1930s. At that time, Japanese cultivators began growing mushrooms on logs wrapped in rice straw. The farmer would find a log with reishi or shiitake growing on it, cut a slice from the log, and sandwich the log between other logs. Then the farmer would bind all the logs in rice straw. Soon the spores from the infected log would infect the other logs as well and mushrooms would begin growing on all the logs.

The log method of cultivating mushrooms worked very well, but then farmers hit on the idea of burying an infected log in the soil. With this technique, the log retained moisture longer, which encouraged the mushrooms to grow. What's more, the log wasn't exposed to and infected by unwanted weed fungi. Another cultivation method is to place mycelium from a mushroom on a wooden plug, drill a small hole in a log, hammer the plug into the log, and wax over the small hole to keep foreign spores out.

Recently, with the popularity of mushrooms on the rise and demand for mushrooms at an all-time high, cultivators have sought more advanced techniques for controlled cultivation. One technique is to cultivate the mushrooms in sawdust. This way, the fruit-bodies of the shiitake mushroom, for example, grown in ninety days, whereas cultivating the mushroom on logs requires eighteen months.

Another technique is to cultivate the mushrooms on grains such as brown rice, barley, or buckwheat. The grains are sterilized and placed into special bags that allow the mycelium to breathe but keep contaminants out. The pristine environment is essential. By the end of the growth cycle, the mycelium has eaten the grain and digested it. As long as the grower's technique is good, very little of the grain remains intact.

In Asia, where demand for medicinal mushroom products is especially high and the products are produced en masse, growers have been devising state-of-the-art techniques to cultivate mycelium. One technique is to grow the mycelium in a liquid culture. Mushroom cultures are introduced into a liquid broth. The growers are quite secretive about their techniques, but suffice it to say, the culture is harvested from the liquid medium and dried into a powder.

Mycologists and growers often tout the superior qualities of the strains they produce. A mushroom *strain* is a culture from a particular mushroom. Mycologists obtain mushroom strains in various ways. The majority purchase them from a mycological culture bank such as the one run by American Type Culture Collection, a company that provides biological products to science and industry. Mycologists often trade cultures among themselves. Many have large collections in libraries. Diligent and meticulous mycologists, however, prefer to obtain the strains from mushrooms they collect themselves in the wild. These mycologists, who strive for the highest-quality mushroom, believe that seeing a mushroom in its native environment and acquainting yourself with its special features is essential. Where a mushroom grows, how quickly it grows, and its virulency matter.

Controlled Cultivation and Analytical Chemistry

Mushroom cultivation has reached new heights of sophistication in recent years, with producers going to great lengths to replicate the growing environment of mushrooms in the laboratory. For example, the *Cordyceps* species, *Cordyceps sinensis* included, is found in oxygen-deficient environments. *Cordyceps* grows in the Himalayas, in swampy areas where high levels of methane and carbon dioxide are found, and in valleys around volcanoes. Because *Cordyceps* grows in these oxygen-deficient environments, it must use oxygen in a very efficient manner. Some mycologists , experimenting with *Cordyceps* in their laboratories, discovered that they could produce higher quantities of cordycepin by depriving *Cordyceps* mycelium of a certain amount of oxygen. Cordycepin is used to treat bacterial infections such as tuberculosis and leprosy, as well as HIV replication. By altering the growing parameters with temperature-gas mixes and nutrient mixes, these mycologists can produce target compounds more efficiently than can be produced with random growth patterns.

The mushroom-growing industry has devoted itself almost exclusively to producing larger fruit-bodies and consistent crops of mushroom fruit-bodies. Not many producers have turned their attention to producing chemical compounds from mushrooms. When mycologists experiment with producing compounds in their mushrooms, they change the growth parameters and got some odd-looking fruit-bodies. These mushrooms would not be marketable in the culinary market as shiitakes, for instance, because they're ugly and pink. But that's okay because mycologists are not looking for a good strain to market. They are trying to produce Lentinan, Krestin, Cordycepin, and other compounds more efficiently.

The past twenty years have seen real advancements in the field of analytical chemistry, and some mycologists have brought these advancements to bear on the cultivation and study of medicinal mushrooms. In a nutshell, analytical chemistry is trying to see how things fit together that are too small to see. Gas chromatography, liquid chromatography, X-ray diffraction, nuclear magnetic resonance (NMR), and other advancements in the field of analytical chemistry have made it possible to see compounds that couldn't be seen before. Each of these methods uses slightly different computerized technology to look at the structure and constituents of molecules. In gas chromatography, for example, scientists place a substance in an extremely low vacuum and blast it apart into fragments. Then, similar to forensic experts piecing together the debris of a bomb blast, the scientists look at the molecular fragments and reassemble them to find out how they were put together before the blast.

Mycologists can use advanced techniques in analytical chemistry to quickly, accurately, and relatively inexpensively test the compounds in mushrooms. They can find out what these compounds are with a degree of certainty never known before. For that matter, they can discover new compounds. The new technologies will be especially useful in the emerging field of mapping beta glucan structures. What was assumed in the past can actually be quantified. These are indeed exciting days in the field of medicinal mushrooms. We can expect to discover new compounds, some of which will serve to prevent or cure disease, in the years ahead.

Cultivating Mycelium in the Laboratory

Using cell-culture technology, it is now possible to grow mushroom mycelium in the laboratory (the mycelium is the feeding body of the mushroom that grows beneath the soil). The processes for growing mycelium are very technical, but suffice it to say that the mycelium is produced in much the same way that baker's and brewer's yeasts are produced. Given the right environment and conditions, mycelium made in the laboratory has the same biological activity as mycelium that is grown in the wild. What's more, it is cleaner and more potent. The electronically controlled culture systems keep out foreign contaminant, and ensure that natural constituents are kept at optimum levels.

Recently, scientists Dr. Randy Dorian of Hanuman Medical of San Francisco and Dr. Moshe Shifrine of Santa Fe, New Mexico, succeeded beyond the wildest dreams of professional mycologists by cultivating truffles (*Tuber melasporum*) in liquid culture. The scientists used mammalian cell tissue culturing techniques to grow fungal tissue. Their success was verified through DNA analysis. Many mycologists are still shaking their heads in awe of this heretofore impossible feat. Truffles contain many interesting compounds that may have significant value for the nutriceutical industry.

From the health-conscious consumer's point of view, maybe the best thing about laboratory-produced mycelium is its cost. *Cordyceps* mushrooms, for example, cost as much as $1,000 per kilo. By contrast, most pharmacies and health food stores sell a *Cordyceps* powder that is significantly less expensive than that. Mushrooms and mushroom products that only the nobility could afford three hundred years ago are now available to everyone. We expect mushroom products to be available in supermarkets soon, as the popularity of the products is increasing.

Shopping for Mushroom Products

Anyone who shops for mushrooms or mushroom products must be aware that some products are better than others. The last decade or so has seen a large increase in the number of mushroom farms, especially in the northwestern United States where the climate is damp and conducive to growing mushrooms. On some occasions, the people who manage these farms, while well intentioned, produce mushrooms of inferior quality because they start from weak isolates. The problem is that most of the mushrooms are grown from hybridized strains and these strains have only a five- to eight-year lifespan. After that, they weaken and their bioefficiency drops out.

It's as simple as this: The grower gets the mushroom strain from a supplier and reproduces it. At first the growing is successful, but the success rate will decline unless the grower knows how to maintain the strain under laboratory conditions. That is a delicate matter requiring more expertise than most people can lay claim to. We have observed that books about cultivating mushrooms usually offer advice for growing or harvesting, but offer little in the way of how to maintain the original fungus, and that is the crucial issue. In the future, we hope that organizations that present mushroom-growing seminars to amateur mycologists will include in-depth training in long-term culture maintenance.

Because temperature and climate are so important in mushroom cultivation, Japanese suppliers have been creating strains especially for use in different climates. In Kyushu Province, where it is warmer, one strain is used; in the northern, colder part of the country, growers use a different strain. Different strains for different climates is nothing new in the world of agriculture. After all, strains of apple, cherry, and all other fruit trees are planted where they will grow best. However, many American mushroom growers are not as sophisticated as they could be. They are not taking climate into account.

Another thing for consumers of mushroom products to consider is how the mycelium is handled. As Chapter One in this book explains, the mycelium is the feeding body of the mushroom that grows underground. Preferably, mushroom mycelium should be processed from start to finish on the same site. Mushroom mycelium is a fragile substance. When it is jostled about or moved from place to place, it can be shocked and bruised, which inhibits its healthy growth cycle. The ideal mycelium mushroom product is harvested at the peak of its vigor and processed immediately on site.

Mushrooms are great absorbers. Like sponges, they take in what is in their environment. Growers who adhere to organic growing procedures produce mushrooms of the highest purity. For that reason, mushroom products that originate in the United States are preferable to mushroom products that originate in industrialized areas in other parts of the planet, where pollution and environmental toxins are often more prevalent.

A Word about Prices

As a raw material, medicinal mushrooms are more expensive than most of the other herbal supplements that you can buy in health food stores. The price of a quality medicinal mushroom product runs between twelve and a hundred dollars for a one-month supply, depending on the quality and number of strains in the formula. If you encounter a mushroom product that costs less than ten dollars, you should be wary. As they become popular, more and more mushroom products are appearing on the market, and some of these products are of inferior quality. Please be careful. The producers of mushroom products who are listed and described in this book have been chosen for their reliability and long, successful track record of supplying quality products. They represent the highest quality and value for your dollar. Before you purchase a medicinal mushroom product, do your homework and find the one from which you will obtain the most health benefits. Unfortunately, but very likely, that product will cost more than twelve dollars.

Mushrooms in the Mainstream

Several years ago, Andrew Miller, a co-author of this book, began experimenting with extracts from reishi fruit-bodies in the course of producing herbal sparkling wines in California's Napa Valley. Miller decided to see what would happen if he blended mediocre red table wine and red reishi fruit-body extracts. The idea was to see if he could make a tonic wine. Miller's company, Tonic Wines and Beers, Inc., already made a ginseng champagne, a blend of high-quality Napa Valley *methode champenoise* and wild American ginseng. His ginseng champagne proved a resounding success and received much critical acclaim from winemakers who had previously been skeptical.

The reishi–red wine blend, a mix of a *cardiotonic*—a substance that strengthens the heart—and "the mushroom of immortality," turned out to be a happy marriage. The wine had an unusual silky texture that fooled Miller's friends in the winemaking industry, who thought they were drinking a top-drawer Napa Valley red. Curiously, Miller's application to produce and sell the unusual new wine was rejected by the Bureau of Alcohol, Tobacco, and Firearms (ATF). The bureau noted that the reishi mushroom is not on the Food and Drug Administration's official list of herbs that can be added to alcoholic beverages, and it rejected Miller's request. Undaunted, Miller continues his work with marrying tonic herbs with wine and is achieving many interesting results.

Recently, bakers in San Francisco's Bay Area have begun experimenting with the use of medicinal-mushroom mycelium cultivated on whole grains. The mycelium powder can be blended in flour and used in baking. As the whole-grain mycelium is heated during the baking process, its beta glucans become more bioavailable. In other words, they are made easier to digest. Putting whole-grain mushroom mycelium in baked goods is a novel and effective way to take the mushrooms, especially where children are concerned, since youngsters often balk at taking pills and capsules. On many occasions we have put reishi and *Agaricus blazei* mycelium powder in our families' pancake mix without anyone being the wiser.

Contemporary cuisine has begun to make use of culinary mushrooms. Oyster mushrooms (*Pleurotus ostreatus*), maitakes, Pom Pom Blancs (*Hericium erinaceus*), and *Agaricus blazei* are now showing up in the kitchens of some of America's best chefs. Apart from their medicinal value, these mushrooms are delicious. They are often the defining element in the dish in which they are served. Savvy chefs are proudly pointing out to their clientele that they are getting something rare and valuable—a food item that has been revered since ancient times for its flavor, as well as its health-giving properties.

Now that the general public in the United States and other formerly mycophobic countries are beginning to embrace mushrooms, we hope to see more mushrooms in the diet, and, dare we say it, more mushroom additives in food. Recently, a fungus-based meat substitute marketed under the brand name Quorn has appeared on the shelves of some markets. Quorn has been popular in Europe for some time and recently received FDA approval in the United States. The product, made from the fungus *Fusarium venenatum,* is supposed to taste, of course, like chicken.

The Story of the Orgasmic Mushroom

To make sure that this book is not anticlimactic, we offer the story of the orgasmic mushroom, a mushroom of the genus *Dictyophora.* This mushroom has not been granted GRAS (Generally Recognized as Safe) status by the United States' Food and Drug Administration. It has not been clinically tested. Some of what we are about to report about the mushroom is highly speculative, but we believe our curious readers would like to know.

Mushrooms of the genus *Dictyophora* do not have aerial spore bodies. Similar to plants, they depend on insects to reproduce. The insects are attracted by the odor of the mushroom. They come to the mushroom, get its sticky spores on their bodies, and carry off the spores. As the insects travel from place to place, they spread the *Dictyophora*'s spores and ensure its survival.

On the Big Island of Hawaii, on the hot, rocky lava flows, there grows a unique species of *Dictyophora* mushroom. The mushroom has a very fast life cycle, even faster than most *Dictyophora*s. It lives between thirty minutes and four hours. Consequently, the mushroom has a very pungent odor. It needs a strong odor to attract insects—and thereby reproduce—during its short lifespan. Researchers have discovered that insect behavior is dictated by the sense of smell and that sex pheromones in plant odors are what attract insects to plants. Mushrooms of the genus *Dictyophora* smell something like rotting meat. They give off a strong odor due to a large number of sex pheromones. Mycologists report that you can smell the mushroom from thirty feet away.

It is believed that the *Dictyophora* species that grows in Hawaii produces a compound that is identical to or a very close mimic of the compound that is produced in human females during the arousal stage. How this compound works in the human female can be described in terms of neurotransmitters. These are chemicals, produced in the brain or elsewhere in the body, that create activity in the brain. For example, when you are frightened, the body creates a small amount of adrenaline and it has a profound and nearly instant effect. Adrenaline is a potent neurotransmitter. Similarly, in the human female, a compound, unnamed as yet, is emitted during arousal. As a woman goes through the various stages of arousal, the level of this compound increases in her blood. Eventually, it reaches a threshold quantity, at which point a cascade of physical events is triggered—an orgasm.

When you cut your arm, your brain produces small amounts of what is essentially morphine, the same chemical compound that the opium poppy produces. Just as poppies produce morphine millions of times greater than what the brain requires, the species of *Dictyophora* in question produces a compound millions of times greater than a woman produces naturally in her body during arousal. The compound is a volatile one. When a woman smells one of these mushrooms, a spontaneous, intense orgasm may occur. The species of *Dictyophora* found in Hawaii has become quite popular with some mycologists for that very reason.

Phallus impudicus, the "orgasm mushroom," is nothing new and enjoys a rich folklore in many lands. A glance at the genus may explain where its reputation comes from. The mushroom resembles a phallus. Hadrianus Junius, in his *Phalli: A Description with Pictures from Life of the Fungi Growing Occasionally in the Sand in Holland*, wrote the following about the mushroom in the sixteenth century: "[It] is very effective for intense and unbearable pains in the joints, above all those caused by passions and limitless debaucheries that exceed the limits of license."

The mushroom is used in New Guinea to encourage cattle to breed. In traditional Chinese medicine, it is used to relieve rheumatism. It is a folk remedy for ulcers, asthma, gout, and other ailments in Latvia. In England, the mushroom is known by the names Stinkhorn, Devil's Stinkpot, Devil's Horn, Stinking Polecat, and Wood Witch.

In her memoir *Period Piece*, Gwen Raverat (1885–1957) writes the following about her Aunt Etty, a proper Victorian lady who took it upon herself to remove the gaudy Stinkhorn mushroom from the nearby woods to protect young ladies' morals. By the way, the Aunt Etty in this passage was the daughter of none other than Charles Darwin. The Latin "grosser name" she refers to, you will recall, is *Phallus impudicus.*

> In our native woods there grows a kind of toadstool, called in the vernacular The Stinkhorn, though in Latin it bears a grosser name. This name is justified for the fungus can be hunted by the scent alone; and this was Aunt Etty's greatest invention: armed with a basket and a pointed stick, and wearing a special hunting cloak and gloves, she would sniff her way round the wood, pausing here and there, her nostrils twitching, when she caught whiff of her prey; then at last, with a deadly pounce, she would fall upon her victim, and then poke his putrid carcass into her basket. . . . The catch was brought back and burnt in deepest secrecy on the drawing-room fire, with all the doors locked, because of the morals of the maids!

Mycologists believe that the *Dictyophora* species that grows on the lava flows of the Big Island of Hawaii, because it lives in such a harsh environment, has evolved an especially intense odor. Very few insects live on the lava flows. To call flies and other insects from a distance, the odor must be especially pungent and the compound that produces the odor must be especially strong.

By some estimates, as many as fifty percent of American woman suffer from *orgasmic dysfunction,* which is defined as difficulty achieving orgasm or the inability to achieve orgasm. Scientists hope to isolate the compound in the *Dictyophora* species from Hawaii and make it available to these women. One problem will be devising test protocols for experimental trials. Telling subjects that they are being tested to see if they achieve states of arousal or orgasms is almost guaranteed to skew the test results. One proposed technique is to take saliva swabs from subjects in the nonaroused state and at different stages of arousal, run the samples through a gas chromatograph, and note how the "arousal compound" increases in intensity after the *Dictyophora*-derived substance is administered.

Incidentally, the mushroom does not appear to be effective in men. Men find the odor of *Dictyophora* nothing short of repulsive. A handful of male scientists, however, in an attempt to answer the age-old question of what an orgasm feels like to women, have proposed giving the mushroom compound to men in quantities high enough to trigger a female orgasm.

The Value of Multiple-Mushroom Formulas

Anyone who goes to the health food store in search of mushroom products inevitably finds what the health food industry calls "multiple-mushroom formulas." Each formula is a mixture of three to as many as fourteen different mushrooms in powder form. The idea is to cover as many bases as possible in a single formula. Reishi, shiitake, *Cordyceps,* and other medicinal mushrooms each offer different health benefits. The different polysaccharide structures in the different mushrooms trigger different receptors of the immune system. The idea is to feed the body a lot of different polysaccharide structures to brighten or lift its immune system relatively quickly.

As Chapter Two explains, each mushroom appears to produce its own unique type of beta glucan. One may stimulate the production of T cells while another helps natural killer cells do their job. *Agaricus blazei,* for example, stimulates the production of natural killer cells. Maitake stimulates the production of T cells. By putting both mushrooms in the mix, you stimulate T and natural killer cells.

It is nearly impossible to tell which part of the immune system fails when a tumor, for example, starts growing uncontrollably. Multiple-mushroom formulas take the shotgun approach. Because each kind of mushroom produces a slightly different 1-3 beta glucan, each mushroom in the formula can aid the immune system in a different way.

Incidences of anyone having a reaction to a medicinal mushroom are very, very rare. Usually, when someone has a bad reaction, the cause is a lack of an enzyme for digesting a particular mushroom. Very few anaphylactic reactions have ever been recorded when taking medicinal mushrooms. For these reasons, mixing many kinds of mushrooms into a formula is safe.

The most sophisticated and advanced multi-mushroom formula of which the authors are aware is called Nikken Bio-Directed Immunity. The formula combines fourteen different medicinal mushrooms, including the eight described in this book. The product is sold and distributed by Nikken, a worldwide distributor of health-related products. If you prefer to take a so-called multiple-mushroom formula, you owe it to yourself to read the label to find out how much of each mushroom is in the formula. Also note what percentage of the formula is composed of each mushroom. The "Producers List" near the end this book lists companies that offer multiple-mushroom formulas.

Trial of a Six-Mushroom Formula

Researchers in the United States along with Chinese scientists Wang Ruwei, Xu Yiyuan, Ji Peijun, and Wang Xingli, conducted a clinical trial with a multi-mushroom formula in People's Hospital of Lishui City, Zhejiang Province, China. The formula consisted of powder in tablet form from six mushrooms: *Agaricus blazei*, shiitake, maitake, reishi, *Trametes versicolor*, and *Cordyceps sinensis*. The study was conducted on fifty-six patients in the middle to late stages (Stage 3 and 4) of cancer. In terms of their physical condition, white blood cell count, granular leukocyte count, and appetite, the subjects of the study were similar. Thirty patients were given 6 grams per day of the multiple-mushroom formula; twenty-six patients were given 30 milligrams a day of the pharmaceutical drug Polyactin-A. Rather than give the comparison group a placebo, as is the custom in the West, Chinese physicians prefer to give the comparison group a medicine. Although this makes the results of experiments harder to assess, Chinese physicians believe for ethical reasons that giving comparison groups some kind of treatment is necessary. All patients in the study were treated concurrently with radiotherapy or chemotherapy a week after they began taking either the multiple-mushroom formula or Polyactin-A. Both groups took their medications for a total of two months.

At the end of the trial period, the multiple-mushroom group showed improvements beyond those of the comparison group. The scientists wrote about their study, "It was shown that the mixed polysaccharides can inhibit the protein synthesis of cancer cells, change the physiological condition of cancer cells, inhibit the growth and transference of cancer cells, relieve the poisoning action of anticancer drugs, improve the patients' sleep and appetite, and result in overall improvement of the symptoms." The scientists concluded that the curative effect of the multiple-mushroom formula was higher than that of Polyactin A and that it can serve a helper role in the treatment of tumor patients.

Multiple Mushrooms (Maitake, Shiitake) and High Blood Pressure

Nothing improves with age except great Bordeaux wines. As we grow older, we are more likely to suffer from high blood pressure, or *hypertension*. The disorder is caused by tension, or pressure, on the arteries that constricts the flow of blood and makes the heart work harder. The causes of hypertension are hard to pinpoint. Most people inherit the disorder from their parents—in other words, hypertension is genetic. Corpulence, poor diet, lack of exercise, and environmental factors can also play a role. Many researchers believe that stress contributes to high blood pressure. Interestingly, the disorder is much more prevalent in industrialized societies than underdeveloped ones.

When the heart beats, a surge of blood is pumped through the arteries of the heart. Blood pressure readings comprise two numbers. The first and higher number, your *systolic* blood pressure, measures the pressure on your arteries as the heart contracts and blood pushes against the artery walls. The second and lower number, your *diastolic* blood pressure, measures the pressure on your arteries when the heart relaxes between beats. The desirable blood pressure reading is 120/80.

In what amounted to an experiment with multiple-mushroom formulas, researchers at Tohoku University in Japan experimented with hypertensive rats to gauge the effect of maitake and shiitake mushrooms on blood pressure. For eight weeks, one group was fed maitake along with its normal diet, another group was fed shiitake, and the third group received no mushroom supplement. After eight weeks, when the groups were compared, researchers discovered that blood pressure in the maitake-fed group had lowered. However, there was no difference between the maitake and control groups in terms of cholesterol levels, triglyceride levels, or plasma levels. (*Plasma* is the portion of the blood that is liquid before clotting; *triglyceride* is a component of the fatty metabolism that is associated with the hardening of the arteries.) By contrast, blood pressure readings were not lower in the shiitake-fed group; however, levels of plasma and triglyceride were lower.

This experiment demonstrates the value of multiple-mushroom formulas. Here, you can see the benefits—in rats, anyway—of taking more than one mushroom. Multiple-mushroom formulas take advantage of the medicinal effects of different mushrooms.

Extract or Capsule Powder?

Essentially, there are three ways to take medicinal mushroom products: as an extract, capsule, or powder. Medicinal mushrooms in capsule form come from dried and powdered mycelium. The mycelium is ground into a powder and encapsulated or pressed into pills. In extract form, water and alcohol are used to extract the active constituents of the mycelium.

Water, for instance, extracts beta glucans (Chapter Two explains what that is). In the case of reishi, alcohol extracts the triterpenes, the element that aids the cardiovascular system. The extract is then bottled and labeled and put on the shelf of health food stores.

Whether you take a mushroom product in extract, capsule, or powder form doesn't matter in terms of the health benefits of the product. What matters is which you are most comfortable taking.

Some companies, such as Garden of Life, Inc. (of Palm Beach Gardens, Florida) believe that predigestion and fermentation of medicinal mushrooms with probiotic cultures—yogurt cultures such as *Lactobacillus acidophilus* and *Bacillus bifidus*—make the mushrooms easier to digest, especially for people whose digestive systems are impaired. All Garden of Life products undergo enzymatic predigestion and lactofermentation. Garden of Life also offers a multiple-mushroom formula called RM-10.

A Word about Cooking Mushrooms

Some of the mushrooms described in this book—maitake and shiitake especially—are very delicious. We encourage you to try your hand at using them in soups, stir-fry dishes, and stews. When you do so, however, be sure to cook them in such a way that they keep their nutrients. The rules that apply to cooking vegetables also apply to cooking mushrooms. If you want to keep the mushrooms' nutrients, you must recover the water in which the mushrooms are cooked. The beta glucan in medicinal mushrooms dissolves into cooking water. Likewise, many nutrients dissolve into the cooking oil when you stir-fry mushrooms. What's more, overcooking depletes the mushrooms of some of their nutrients. The best way to prepare mushrooms is to include the cooking liquids in the dish you are preparing and be careful not to cook the mushrooms for too long. Some connoisseurs believe in tearing mushrooms instead of cutting them to preserve nutrients. By tearing, the mushrooms pieces are separated along the cell walls.

To clean mushrooms, trim the bottom of the stems and then wipe off the mushrooms. *Do not* soak or rinse them. Mushrooms absorb water; if you wash them in water, your mushrooms will turn soggy and lose some of their crispness and flavor.

Of course, you can always rely on medicinal mushroom powders and capsules to get nutrients from mushrooms. If you prefer not to take powders and capsules, try mixing them into soups or baking them into breads. By the way, mixing medicinal mushroom powders into food is an excellent way to give medicinal mushrooms to children, who often balk at taking pills and capsules.

The Innovators

We thought you might like to go behind the scenes and meet some of the people who produce medicinal mushroom products. In the United States at least, the medicinal mushroom industry—like the herbal medicines industry to which it is related—is fairly new. These pages introduce you to some of the pioneers and innovators of medicinal mushrooms in the United States.

Functional Fungi LLC

Functional Fungi, a California company with production facilities in Arroyo Grande, is being founded for the express purpose of cultivating a variety of medicinal mushroom raw materials for nutriceutical and culinary purposes, all with organic certification. The company's liquid culture mycelial raw materials are the only certified organic variety that we know of. This company is undertaking revolutionary experiments in feeding precursor nutrients to the liquid cultures in which mushrooms grow. A precursor nutrient is a substance or chemical compound that encourages a mushroom or plant to develop in a certain way. The mycologists at Functional Fungi are trying to see if they can make the medicinal compounds in their mushrooms stronger and more potent by sowing precursor nutrients in the substrate that the mushrooms feed on. These potent raw materials are targeted for the nutriceutical as well as the pharmaceutical industry for drug development.

Whereas most companies that produce medicinal mushroom raw materials do so on one type of grain or substrate, this company has experimented with many different grains and grain blends with an eye to finding out how to grow nutrient-rich fungi. This novel approach is based on the age-old idea that a plant is only as good as the soil it grows in.

Functional Fungi's goal is to bring advancements to the art of cultivation and innovation to the range of products currently available to consumers.

John Seleen of MushroomScience

Like many producers in the medicinal mushroom field, John Seleen of MushroomScience LLC, started as a mushroom farmer. For ten years, he grew maitake and shiitake mushrooms for the gourmet market on his farm near Eugene, Oregon. Then, in 1989, John attended a conference in China about advanced cultivation techniques. The conference opened his eyes to the wonders of medicinal mushrooms. John correctly predicted that medicinal mushrooms with their immune-enhancing qualities would find a place in the health-conscious American market. In 1994, he started JHS Natural Products (the precursor to MushroomScience) with the purpose of selling *Trametes versicolor* extracts in the United States. His company was the first to import *Trametes versicolor* extracts chemically matched to the material used in Japanese and Chinese clinical research. Since 1994, MushroomScience has branched out. It now offers *Cordyceps,* maitake, reishi, and *Agaricus blazei* extracts, as well as a multiple-mushroom formula (some of these products are still marketed under the JHS Natural Products label).

What makes MushroomScience stand out is John's commitment to testing and research. MushroomScience maintains a state-of-the-art laboratory where chemists work on refining quality standards. The lab is capable of performing gas chromatography, high-performance liquid chromatography, and proton nuclear magnetic resonance spectroscopy. MushroomScience has customized and formulated an analytical protocol for each extract it produces. The extracts are tested rigorously to maintain high standards. Looking ahead, MushroomScience has been collaborating with a Pennsylvania company to try to improve cultivation techniques and in so doing compete in the marketplace with the inexpensive raw-material mushrooms currently being imported from China.

"Doctors, who are most of our customers, are a tough crowd," said John. "They need to be convinced they should buy a health product. They also want to know how much to prescribe to their patients over what period of time. We look very hard at how to fit our products into the Western pharmacological model. We want our products to have predictable quantities of active compounds so that doctors can do predictable dosing over a long period of time and measure results. You have to speak the language of science to reach the Western market."

John believes that small as well as large producers have an obligation to expand the boundaries of medicinal mushrooms. The company funded a double-blind placebo group study at the National College of Naturopathic Medicine that looked into the use of *Trametes versicolor* extracts to treat hepatitis C. John is happy to report that everyone in the *Trametes* group maintained or improved their health. His company is negotiating with the University of Pittsburgh Cancer Institute on another study that will examine the use of *Trametes versicolor* as a means of treating breast cancer. MushroomScience is collaborating with one of Japan's leading microbial chemists, Dr. Hiroaki Nanba of Kobe Pharmaceutical University, to market Dr. Nanba's newest maitake extract in the United States.

"The benefits of mushrooms aren't limited to the immune system," John said. "They have benefits for cardiovascular health and liver health. They are a great source of protein, essential amino acids, and B vitamins. Medicinal mushrooms are doing a lot of people a lot of good."

Andrew Miller of MycoHerb, Inc.

In 1987, mushroom products were scarce and difficult to find. The only way to find them in the United States was to hunt them down in the Chinatowns of major cities.Convinced of the health benefits of medicinal mushrooms, Andrew Miller, who had been producing herbal products for several years, was determined to make medicinal mushrooms readily available in the United States. In 1987, Miller, along with several mycologically inclined conspirators, including Dr. E. Justin Wilson, a former National Institutes of Health researcher, formed MycoHerb, Inc. The company was a pioneer in producing and marketing medicinal mushroom products.

MycoHerb was the first to use living mycelia to create its products. Under the guiding hand of Dr. Wilson, the company developed a proprietary method for extracting live mycelium. The method captures both water-soluble and alcohol-soluble constituents in a custom-produced, all-glass extraction apparatus. The products are encased in glass at all times so that no valuable oils escape during the creation process. MycoHerb's pioneering techniques have since been copied throughout the industry.

MycoHerb was the first in the United States to produce a line of concentrated liquid extracts from medicinal mushrooms. The company developed a proprietary method for extracting mycelium grown on brown rice. It introduced a liposome delivery spray consisting of a twelve-mushroom formula in 1995. MycoHerb led the way in developing multiple-mushroom formulas. MycoHerb has created many products, including MycoSurge and its liposome delivery system, and continues to be an innovator in the field of medicinal mushroom products.

In the company's early years, when the public did not realize or understand the benefits of medicinal mushrooms, MycoHerb sold its products primarily to health practitioners, doctors, and acupuncturists. Today, MycoHerb products are sold exclusively to health-care practitioners in thirteen countries, including Ireland, the Netherlands, and Denmark, where MycoHerb products have been used as adjunct therapies in hospitals that specialize in the treatment of cancer patients.

Mushrooms and the Connection to the Earth

In the distant human past, all plants and animals were repositories of secret power that could be used for good or ill. In a sense, the whole world was a pharmacopoeia. Our ancestors' relationship to the food they ate was very different from ours. Their food was sacred. They understood nourishment in a different way than we do. Our ancestors believed that the plants and animals they ate were gifts from the divine. Plants and animals had spirits, and when you ate a plant or animal, you partook of its spirit as well.

In our day, most people would have trouble explaining where their food was grown or how it came to the table at which they sit. Too few people appreciate the expertise and effort that goes into cultivating and growing food. We have lost the primal connection to the food we put in our bodies. We have, you could say, not only lost our connection to the food we eat, we have lost our connection to the earth. Most of us understand food in terms of flavor and texture. We don't understand that food is our connection to the earth and its vital energy.

Mushrooms are potent medicines. They contain many nutrients. Mushrooms, which grow so close to the earth, have a grounding effect. When you take a medicinal mushroom product, you get back in touch with the essential forces of the earth. You tap into the sustaining power that incites the animal to endeavor and the plant to grow no matter what the obstacle. Humankind has been nourished by medicinal mushrooms for many centuries. We look forward with great enthusiasm to new discoveries by which modern science will harness mushrooms' medicinal power for the good of humankind in the years to come.

Recipes for Mushroom Dishes

We would like to thank Malcolm Clark for offering these recipes for mushroom dishes. Not all the recipes here call for the medicinal mushrooms described in this book, but feel free to experiment by substituting your favorite mushrooms for the ones listed in these recipes.

Gourmet Mushroom Pot Pie

Serves six

This is a simple but delicious recipe that can be made a day or two ahead if desired. Any combination of mushrooms can be used. I always like to include some dry mushrooms such as shiitake or porcini because they have much more intense flavor than their fresh counterparts.

2 tablespoons *each* unsalted butter and olive oil

$\frac{1}{4}$ cup chopped shallots or green onions

1 tablespoon minced garlic

$\frac{1}{2}$ ounce dried porcini, softened in warm water, drained and chopped

3 cups shiitake mushrooms, stems removed and thickly sliced

3 cups mixed gourmet mushrooms, cleaned and halved (Trumpet Royal, Clamshell, Namkeo)

3 cups oyster mushrooms, stems removed and separated

$\frac{1}{2}$ cup dry white wine

$1\frac{1}{2}$ cups rich chicken or vegetable stock

2 tablespoons Dijon mustard

$1\frac{1}{2}$ cups heavy cream

2 teaspoons chopped fresh thyme (teaspoon dried)

Salt and freshly ground black pepper

Softened butter for pot pie dishes

Herbed bread crumbs (recipe below)

Add the butter and oil to a large sauté pan along with the shallots and garlic and sauté over moderate heat until softened but not brown. Add the mushrooms and increase heat and sauté until lightly colored. Add the next six ingredients and simmer for five minutes. Strain the mixture and set the mushroom mixture aside. Retrun sauce to pan and reduce over high heat by half to a medium sauce consistency (about ten minutes).

Stir mushrooms back into sauce and season to taste with salt and pepper. Divide among six lightly buttered one-cup ovenproof pot pie dishes. Sprinkle herb bread crumb mixture on top of each and place in a hot oven so that mushrooms are bubbling and topping is lightly browned. Serve immediately.

Note: If making ahead, be sure to refrigerate pot pies and add crumb mixture just before they go into the oven.

Herb Bread Crumb Crust

¾ cup coarse white bread crumbs (Japanese panko prefered)

¾ cup freshly grated Asiago or Parmesan cheese

¼ cup fresh chopped parsley

2 tablespoons finely chopped fresh chives

1 tablespoon finely chopped fresh basil

1 teaspoon finely grated lemon zest

Drops of olive oil

Combine all ingredients in a bowl with a few drops of olive oil to very lightly coat. Set aside until ready to use.

> *Recommended wine:* Mushrooms and Merlot or Pinot Noir are a great match.

Exotic Mushroom Frittata

Preheat oven to 325°

1 medium onion, diced

1 clove garlic, minced

8 ounces fresh exotic mushrooms, finely diced (exotic mushroom choices: shiitake, Clamshell, Trumpet Royal)

3 tablespoons olive oil

6 eggs, beaten

¼ cup bread crumbs

¼ teaspoon salt

⅛ teaspoon each: oregano, white pepper, Tabasco

½ pound Monterey Jack cheese, grated

2 tablespoons finely chopped fresh cilantro

Sauté onion, garlic, and exotic mushrooms in olive oil, over medium heat, until barely limp. Add beaten eggs. Combine all remaining ingredients, mixing well. Turn into buttered 7- x 11-inch pan. Bake for about thirty minutes or until firm and lightly browned. Cool and cut into one-inch squares.

Makes about 6 dozen 1-inch squares.

Gourmet Mushroom Chowder

Serves six

4 cups sliced onions

2 tablespoons butter

$1/2$ pound mixed gourmet mushrooms (Brown Clamshell, Alba Clamshell, Blue Oyster, Black Oyster, sliced Trumpet Royal)

2 tablespoons flour

4 cups warm chicken stock or fish stock

4 cups sliced boiling potatoes

Herb bouquet (four parsley sprigs, $1/2$ bay leaf preferably imported, $1/2$ cup thyme)

Optional: three medium chicken breasts; or 6 boneless chicken thighs, cooked and slivered; or 1 to $1^{1/2}$ pounds fish filets, cut into chunks

$1/2$ cup sour cream

Sauté four cups of sliced onions in two tablespoons of butter. When tender but not browned, add the mushrooms and sauté for two minutes. Blend in two tablespoons of flour and cook slowly for two minutes; then remove from heat and blend in, by dribbles at first, four cups of chicken or fish stock. Add four cups of sliced potatoes and an herb bouquet, and simmer fifteen to twenty minutes, or until the potatoes are tender. Taste, and add salt and pepper as needed.

You can also use fish instead of chicken, but replace the chicken stock with fish stock. Serve in big soup bowls and accompany with Pilot crackers or fresh French bread.

Coconut Soup with Gourmet Mushrooms (*Tom Kha Gai*)

Serves four

1 cup coconut milk, divided

1 cup chicken stock

6 thin slices ginger

½ teaspoon fresh chopped jalapeño chili

2 stalks lemon grass/citronella, lower ½ portion only, cut into one-
inch lengths and crushed

5 fresh basil leaves

½ boned chicken breast, sliced

5 tablespoons fish sauce

8 ounces mixed gourmet mushrooms (use a combination of Alba
Clam Shell, Brown Clam Shell, Nameko, and sliced Trumpet
Royal)

1 tablespoon sugar

½ cup lime juice

¼ cup cilantro/coriander leaves, torn

Combine half the coconut milk and the chicken stock with the ginger, lemon grass, and basil leaves in a large saucepan and heat to boiling. Add the chicken, fish sauce, mushrooms, and sugar. Simmer for about four minutes or until the chicken is cooked. Add the remaining coconut milk to the saucepan and heat just to boiling. Place the lime juice and chili paste in a serving bowl and then pour the soup into the serving bowl. Garnish with the torn cilantro leaves and crushed chili peppers, and serve.

Gourmet Mushroom Tapenade

I love this concoction, which is a delicious condiment on almost anything. I use it to make vegetarian sushi or as a topping on bruschetta. It's also great on simply grilled or broiled fish, shellfish, and chicken.

Makes approximately 1¼ cups

¼ cup finely chopped white onion

2 teaspoons finely chopped garlic

2 teaspoons minced fresh peeled ginger

4 tablespoons canola or grapeseed oil

½ pound shiitake or gourmet mushrooms (Trumpet Royal, Clamshell, Nameko), stems removed and cut into ¼-inch dice

2 tablespoons reduced-salt soy sauce

3 tablespoons seasoned rice vinegar

1 teaspoon hot pepper sesame oil (or to taste)

⅛ teaspoon five-spice powder

2 teaspoons fresh lemon juice

1 teaspoon chopped, rinsed salted black beans (optional)

1 tablespoon chopped cilantro

Sauté the onion, garlic, and ginger in two tablespoons of oil until softened but not brown. Set aside to cool. Add remaining two tablespoons oil to a pan and sauté mushrooms quickly until just beginning to brown (sauté in batches with a little more oil, if necessary). Add mushrooms to onion mixture and stir in remaining ingredients. Store covered in refrigerator up to one week.

Bruschetta with Gourmet Mushrooms

4 tablespoons olive oil

1 large shallot, minced

2 tablespoons chopped parsley

1½ pounds mixed gourmet mushrooms (shiitake, Trumpet Royale, Black
  Oyster, Blue Oyster, or Chanterelle), cleaned and sliced

Salt and pepper

6 slices country-style bread, ½-inch thick

½ cup olive oil

1 large garlic clove, peeled

Heat a large skillet over high heat. Coat the pan with olive oil. Add shallots, garlic, and parsley and cook until shallots are soft. Add mushrooms and cook until they begin to brown. Adjust seasoning with salt and pepper.

Toast bread over a hot grill or under a broiler. Brush with olive oil and rub with the garlic clove while still hot. Top with sautéed mushrooms and serve with a glass of Chardonnay.

Fabulous Porcini Risotto for Two

1 tablespoon dried porcini powder

6 pieces sliced porcini (optional but desirable)

Pinch of sugar

4 tablespoons butter or olive oil

3/4 cup dry white wine

2 tablespoons grated Parmigiano-Reggiano

1 teaspoon porcini oil

2 cups chicken stock

1 cup porcini stock

3/4 cup Arborio rice

Prepare porcini stock by placing one tablespoon dry porcini powder, sliced porcini, and a pinch of sugar in one cup warm water. Let soak for thirty to sixty minutes (for the well organized: cover overnight in the refrigerator).

Take the sliced porcini in your hand and squeeze out the liquid. Set porcini aside with the rice. Mix porcini stock and chicken stock together in a saucepan and heat to almost a simmer.

Rice Preparation

Melt two tablespoons butter or oil in a saucepan. When good and hot, add the rice and sliced porcini (first-time risotto makers set your clocks for twenty minutes). Stir continually and cook for approximately one minute on medium heat.

Add the dry white wine. Stir and simmer down until almost all the liquid has gone. Add one cup of prepared stock. Simmer down again (the starch should be really coming out now). Repeat twice again using all the stock (three times).

When the liquid has almost gone on the third time, add the remaining two table-spoons of butter/oil and two tablespoons grated cheese. Mix briskly for one minute; then turn off the heat. Add one teaspoon or more to taste of porcini oil to the mixture and serve immediately. Bite a piece of rice to test if done, or slice a few grains in half. They should be soft going to firm with a pinprick of white in the center (al dente). Cooking takes approximately twenty minutes with the recommended portions; a truly al dente finish is expected.

To prepare for four or more diners, keep doubling the ingredients and allow a little more time. Risotto gets better with practice and you can make slight variations according to your own taste.

PRODUCERS LIST

Medicinal mushroom products can be found in many pharmacies, health-food stores, Chinese herb stores, and on the Internet. But if you have difficulty finding the medicinal mushroom you're looking for, the following list will guide you to a producer or supplier who can sell the mushroom product to you directly or inform you of the nearest retail outlet. We can vouch for the following companies. They offer the best, highest-quality medicinal mushroom products on the market.

Atlas World USA, Inc.
444 South Flower Street
Suite 1650
Los Angeles, CA 90071
Tel: 213/627-3430
Fax: 213/689-9499
Web site: www.AtlasWorldUSA.com
Products: *Agaricus blazei,* maitake, shiitake

This company offers some of the best and most thoroughly researched *Agaricus blazei* products on the market. The company provides a health supplement called Agaricus Bio, a face cream called Radiance, and a health supplement for pets called Immune Booster. Atlas World, Japan, Inc. was founded in Tokyo in 1995. The company's goal is to produce the highest-quality *Agaricus blazei* products and it has certainly done that. Atlas World USA, Inc. was founded to cultivate *Agaricus blazei* in the United States. The company's products are made with a proprietary formula in which *Agaricus blazei* from all four stages of the mushroom's life cycle—the spore, mycelium, primordia, and fruit-body stage—are used (the primordia stage, also called the "pinhead" stage, describes when the fruit-body first emerges). Melissa Northway, Atlas's enthusiastic and hardworking marketing director, tells us that the company's *Agaricus blazei* products are made from all four stages to get the most potency from the mushroom. The company has a patent pending on its *Agaricus blazei* cream for protection against ultraviolet B rays.

Elixir
8612 Melrose Ave.
Los Angeles, CA 90069
Tel: 310/657-9300
Web site: www.Elixir.net
Products: Multiple-mushroom formula

This company, a favorite of Hollywood glitterati, offers a product called Mushroom Resistance Tonic, a blend of reishi, maitake, and shiitake mushrooms.

Functional Fungi LLC
P.O. Box 68
Arroyo Grande, CA 93421
Web site: www.FunctionalFungi.com
E-mail: sales@functionalfungi.com

This California company is raising the bar on quality and innovation in the cultivation of medicinal mushrooms. A wide range of species, including *Cordyceps sinensis* and *Agaricus blazei,* are available as mycelium. The mushrooms are produced through an advanced technology for optimizing nutrients. The company also produces products derived from liquid-culture technology. Based in Arroyo Grande, California, this company specializes in providing certified-organic raw materials to nutriceutical and pharmaceutical manufacturers and is active in the development of functional foods created from and delivering the benefits of medicinal and nutritional mushrooms.

Garden of Life, Inc.
1449 Jupiter Park Drive
Suite 16
Jupiter, FL 33458
Tel: 800/622-8986
FAX: 561/575-5488
Web site: www.GardenofLifeUSA.com
Products: Multiple-mushroom formulas

This company provides a multiple-mushroom formula called RM-10 that includes many of the mushrooms described in this book: reishi, shiitake, *Cordyceps, Hericium erinaceus,* and others. The company specializes in probiotics that benefit the gastrointestinal tract. RM-10 is being studied for its effects on the immune system and the five most common cancers at Bio-Inova Laboratories in Plaisir, France. The product will be the subject of a seventy-patient clinical study on chronic fatigue syndrome being conducted in the United States. All results will be published in peer-review journals and available to the public in the fall of 2002.

Gourmet Mushrooms, Inc.
2901 Gravenstein Highway
Sebastopol, CA 95472
Tel: 707/823-1743 *or* 707/823-1507
Web site: www.GourmetMushroomsInc.com
Products: Rei-Shi-Gen, a shiitake-reishi combination product

This company is a pioneer in the cultivation of medicinal and culinary mushrooms. The company also provides kits for growing delicious culinary mushrooms.

HYY (BV) Ltd.
Web site: www.houseofyinyang.com/eng/hoyy/product/index.htm
Products: *Trametes versicolor*

This Hong Kong company offers two *Trametes versicolor* health supplements. The supplements, which include PSP (polysaccharopeptide) derived from the COV-1 strain, are called I'm-Yunity and I'm Yunity Too. These supplements offer the *Trametes versicolor* mushroom in capsule form. PSP is probably the most extensively researched mushroom product on the planet.

Marco Pharma International LLC
851 NW Highland Street
Roseburg, OR 97470
Tel: 800/999-3001
Fax: 541/677-8301

This company is the leading specialist in German drainage therapies. Marco Pharma is the exclusive distributor of a twelve-mushroom formula that is delivered through an oral liposome spray technology.

MushroomScience
P.O. Box 50398
Eugene, OR 97405
Tel: 541/344-8753 *or* 888/283-6583
Fax: 541/344-3107
Products: *Cordyceps,* maitake, reishi, and *Agaricus blazei* extracts, as well as a multiple-mushroom formula.

MushroomScience was the first to import *Trametes versicolor* extracts chemically matched to the material used in Japanese and Chinese clinical research. The company has been producing medicinal mushroom products since 1994.

MycoHerb, Inc.
P.O. Box 1844
Burlingame, CA 94011
Tel: 650/343-9840
Fax: 650/434-2704
Products: *Agaricus blazei, Cordyceps sinensis, Hericium erinaceus, Phellinus linteus,* reishi, shiitake, *Trametes versicolor,* multiple-mushroom formulas

This company has been in the nutritive mushroom field since 1987. MycoHerb is one of the few companies that does live culture extraction. Through a proprietary process, lab technicians take the living mushroom biomass and extract its active constituents. MycoHerb provides all the mushrooms covered in this book.

Nikken
Tel: 888/2-NIKKEN
Web site: www.Nikken.com
Products: Multiple-mushroom formula

Nikken, a network marketing company, offers a unique fourteen-mushroom formula that includes several rare species and exclusive strains grown especially for Nikken. Nikken's formula is the Rolls Royce of multiple-mushroom formulas. The global giant, Nikken, is a leader and innovator in the highest quality wellness technology. We strongly recommend checking out the company's Web site.

Planetary Formulas

P.O. Box 553
Soquel, CA 95073
Tel: 831/438-7410
Web site: www.planetaryformulas.com

Planetary Formulas is a northern California-based herbal supplements company providing health food stores and health professionals with Western, Chinese, and Ayurvedic herbal products for more than 20 years. Most products are developed from the more than 30-years clinical experience of world renowned herbalist, author, and acupuncturist, Micheal Tierra, LAc, OMD. Planetary Formulas provides a collection of liquid and tableted single and combination specialty mushroom products including Reishi, Maitake, Shiitake, and Cordyceps. Each is designed to deliver the full spectrum of valuable mushroom constituents in a form that is easily digested and assimilated.

Tea Garden Herbal Emporium

9001 Beverly Blvd.
West Hollywood, CA 90048
Tel: 310/205-0104
Web site: www.TGarden.net
Products: *Cordyceps sinensis,* maitake, reishi, multiple-mushroom formula

This company offers a large line of reishi products, including Wild Reishi Drops, Duanwood Reishi Drops, and Reishi Longevity Elixir.

REFERENCES

Chapter One

Arora, D. 1986. *Mushrooms Demystified.* Berkeley, CA: Ten Speed Press.

Beinfield, H. et al. 1995. Chinese traditional medicine: An introductory overview. *Alternative Therapies.* 1:44–52.

Berman, B et al. 1994. Alternative medicine: Expanding medical horizons: a report to the National Institute of Health on alternative medical systems and practices in the United States. *NIH.* 94–166.

Hobbs, C. 1986. *Medicinal Mushrooms: An Exploration of Tradition, Healing, and Culture.* Santa Cruz, CA: Botanica Press.

Huddler, G. 1998. *Magical Mushrooms, Mischievous Molds.* Princeton, NJ: Princeton Press.

Kaptchuck, T. 2000. *The Web That Has No Weaver: Understanding Chinese Medicine.* Chicago: Contemporary Books.

Keys, J. 1998. *Chinese Herbs: Their Botany, Chemistry, and Pharmacodynamics.* Rutland, VT: Charles E. Tuttle Co.

Nakagaki, T. 2000. Intelligence: Maze-solving by an amoeboid organism. *Nature* 407:123–125.

Reston, J. 1971. Now let me tell you about my appendectomy in Peking. *New York Times* 21 July; 1.

Schaechter, E. 1997. *In the Company of Mushrooms.* Cambridge, MA: Harvard University Press.

Schaechter, E. 2000. Weird and wonderful fungi. *Microbiology Today.* 27:116–117.

Smith, ML et al. 1992. The fungus, *armillaria bulbosa*, is among the largest and oldest living organisms. *Nature.* 356:428–431.

Spindler, K. 1994. *The Man in the Ice: The Discovery of a 5,000-Year-Old Body Reveals the Secrets of the Stone Age.* New York: Bantam Books.

Wasson, R. Gordon. 1968. *The Divine Mushroom of Immortality.* New York: Harcourt Brace Jovanovich.

Yue, D et al. 1995. *Advanced Study for Traditional Chinese Herbal Medicine, Institute of Materia Medica.* Beijing, China: Medical University and China Peking Union Medical University Press.

Chapter Two

Adachi, Y et al. 1994. The effect enhancement of cytokine production by macrophages stimulated with 1,3 beta D glucan, grifolan, isolated from *Grifola frondosa. Biol Pharm Bull.* 17:1554–1560.

Browder, IW et al. 1990. Beneficial effect of enhanced macrophage function in the trauma patients. *Ann Surg.* 211:605–613.

Clute, M. 2001. Beta glucan : The little branched-chain polysaccharide that might. *Natural Foods Merchandiser.* 3:21–24.

DiLuzio, N. 1983. Immunopharmacology of glucan: A broad spectrum enhancer of host defense mechanisms. *Trends Pharmacol.* 4:344–347.

Gibson, G et al. 1995. Dietary modulation of the human colonic microbiota: Introducing the concept of prebiotics. *J Nutr.* 125:1401–1412.

Lewis, R. 2001. Portals for prions? Investigators look at a potential pathway for prions. *The Scientist.* 7:1.

Lui, F. 1997. Free radical scavenging activities of mushroom polysaccharide extracts. *Life Sci.* 60:10:763–771.

Manfreds, D et al. 1992. Morbidity and mortality from chronic obstructive pulmonary disease. *Ann Rev Resp Dis.* 140:S19–S26.

Mansell, PW et al. 1975. Macrophage-mediated destruction of human malignant cells *in vivo. J Natl Cancer Inst.* 54:571–80.

Martensen, R. 1994. Cancer: Medical history and the framing of a disease. *JAMA.* 271:24–28.

Mizuno, T et al. 1995. Health foods and medicinal usage of mushrooms. *Food Rev Intern.* 1:69–81.

Ohno, N et al. 1996. Effect of beta glucan on the nitric oxide synthesis of peritoneal macrophage in mice. *Biol Pharm Bull.* 19:608–612.

Raa, J et al. 1989. The use of immunostimulants to increase resistance of aquatic organisms to microbial infection. *J Dermatol Surg Oncol.* 15:1199–1202.

Rodman, WL. 1893. Cancer, its etiology and treatment. *Am Pract News.* 16:409–417.

Wasser, S. 1999. Medicinal properties of substances occurring in higher basidiomycetes. *Intern J Medicinal Mushr.* 1:31–62.

Chapter Three

Kim, KC et al. 1999. *Ganoderma lucidum* extracts protect DNA from strand breakage caused by hydroxyl radical and UV irradiation. *Int J Mol Med.* 4:273–277.

Wang, SY et al. 1997. The anti-tumor *Ganoderma lucidum* is mediated by cytokines released from activated macrophages and T lymphocytes. *Int J Cancer.* 70:699–705.

Yu, S et al. 2000. An experimental study on the effects of lingzhi spore on the immune function and ^{60}Co radioresistance in mice. *J Nat Prod.* 63(4):514–516.

Zhu, M et al. 1999. Triterpene antioxidants from *Ganoderma lucidum*. *Phytother Res.* 13:529–531.

Chapter Four

Buchwald, D et al. 1996. Functional status in patients with chronic fatigue syndrome, other fatiguing illnesses, and healthy individuals. *Am J Med.* 4:364–370.

Che, YS et al. 1996. Observations on therapeutic effects of jinshuibao on coronary heart disease, hyperlipidemia, and blood rheology. *Chin Trad Herb Dr.* 9:552–553.

Chen, DG. 1995. Effects of jinshuibao capsule on the quality of life of patients with heart failure. *J Admin Tradl Chin Med.*5:40–43.

Clark, AL et al. 1995. The origin of symptoms in chronic heart failure. *Heart.* 5:429–430.

Crouse, SF et al. 1997. Effects of training and single session of exercise on lipids and apolipoproteins in hypercholesterolemic men. *J Appl Physiol.*6:2109–2028.

Fukuda, K et al. 1994. Chronic fatigue syndrome: A comprehensive approach to its definition and study. *Ann Intern Med.* 953–959.

Halpern, GM. 1998. *Cordyceps: China's Healing Mushroom.* New York: Avery Publishing.

Jiang, JC et. al. 1995. Summary of treatment of 37 chronic renal dysfunction patients with jinshuibao. *J Admin Ttradl Chin Med.* 5:23–24.

Kashyap, ML. 1997. Cholesterol and atherosclerosis: A contemporary perspective. *Ann Acad Med Sing.* 4:517–523.

Kennedy, HL. 1997. Beta blockade, ventricular arrhythmias, and sudden cardiac death. *Am J Card.* 9b: 29J–34J.

Lei, M et al. 1995. Jinshubao capsule as adjuvant treatment for acute stage pulmonary heart disease: Analysis of therapeutic effect of 50 clinical cases. *J Adm Trad Chin Med.* 5:28–29.

Lemanske, RF. 1997. Asthma. *JAMA.* 278:1588–1873.

Liu, C et al. 1986. Treatment of 22 patients with post-hepatitis cirrhosis with a preparation of fermented mycelia of *Cordyceps sinensis. Shanghai J Chin Materia Med.* 6:30–31.

Markell, MS. 1997. Herbal therapies and the patient with kidney disease. *Quarter Rev Nat Med.* Fall:189–200.

Pegler, DN et al. 1994. The chinese caterpillar fungus. *The Mycologist.* 8:3–5.

Pereira, J. 1843. Summer-plant-winter-worm. *N Y J Med.* 1:128–132.

Shao, G. et al. 1990. Treatment of hyperlipidemia with *Cordyceps sinensis*: A double-blind placebo-control trial. *Int J Orient Med.* 2:77–80.

Steinkraus, DC et al. 1994. Chinese caterpillar fungus and world record runners. *Am Entomo.* Winter:235–239.

Uoma, PVI et al. 1995. High serum alpha-tocopherol, albumin, selenium, and cholesterol, and low mortality from coronary disease in northern Finland. *J Int Med.* 237:49–54.

Wang, Q et al. 1987. Comparison of some pharmacological effects between *Cordyceps sinensis* and *Cephalosporium sinensis. Bull Chin Mater Med.* 12:682–684.

Xie, FY. 1992. Therapeutic observation of Xingbao in treating 83 patients with asymptomatic hepatitis B. *Chin J Hosp Pharm.* 8:352-353.

Yamaguchi, N et al. 1990. Augmentation of various immune reactivities of tumor-bearing hosts with an extract of *Cordyceps sinensis. Biotherapy 2.* 3:199–205.

Zhang, M et al. 1998. Notes on the alpine *Cordyceps* of China and nearby nations. *Mycotaxon.* 66:215–229.

Zhang, Z et al. 1995. Clinical and laboratory studies of jinshuibao in scavenging oxygen free radicals in elderly senescent xuzheng patients. *J Admin Trad Chin Med.* 5:14–18.

Zhao, CS et al. 2001. CordyMax CS-4 improves glucose metabolism and increases insulin sensitivity in normal rats. In press.

Zhu, JS, Halpern, GM, Jones, K. 1998. The scientific rediscovery of an ancient Chinese herbal medicine: *Cordyceps sinensis. J Altern Compl Med.* 3:239–303.

Chapter Five

Fujimiya, Y et al. 1998. Selective tumoricidal effect of soluble proteoglucan extracted from the basidiomycete, *Agaricus blazei* Murill, mediated via natural killer cell activation and apoptosis. *Cancer Immunol Immunother.* 46:147–159.

Fujimiya, Y et al. 1999. Tumor-specific cytocidal and immunopotentiating effects of relatively low molecular weight products derived from the basidiomycete, *Agaricus blazei* Murill. *Anticancer Res.* 19:113–118.

Ito, H et al. 1997. Anti-tumor effects of a new polysaccharide-protein complex (ATOM) prepared from *Agaricus blazei* (Iwade strain 101) and its mechanisms in tumor-bearing mice. *Anticancer Res.* 17:277–284.

Mizuno, M et al. 1998. Polysaccharides from *Agaricus blazei* stimulate lymphocyte T cell subsets in mice. *Biosci Biotechnol Biochem.* 62:434–437.

Chapter Six

Adachi ,Y et al. 1994. Enhancement of cytokine production by macrophages stimulated with 1-3 beta-D-glucan, grifolan (GRN), isolated from *Grifola frondosa. Biol Pharm Bull.* 17:1554–1560.

Fullerton, SA et al. 2000. Induction of apoptosis in human prostatic cancer cells with beta glucan . *Mol Urol.* 4:7–14.

Kubo, K et al. 1994. Anti-diabetic activity present in the fruit body of *Grifola frondosa* (maitake). *Biol Pharm Bull.* 17:1106–1110.

Kubo, K et al. 1996. The effect of maitake mushrooms on liver and serum lipids. *Altern Ther Health Med.* 2:62–66.

Kurashige, S et al. 1997. Effects of *Lentinus edodes, Grifola frondosa* and *Pleurotus ostreatus* administration on cancer outbreak, and activities of macrophages and lymphocytes in mice treated with a carcinogen, N-butyl-N-butanolnitrosoamine. *Immunopharmacol Immunotoxicol.* 19: 175–183.

Lee, EW et al. 2000. Suppression of D-galactosamine-induced liver injury by mushrooms in rats. *Biosci Biotechnol Biochem.* 64:2001–2004.

Nakai, R et al. 1999. Effect of maitake (*Grifola frondosa*) water extract on inhibition of adipocyte conversion of C3H10T1/2B2C1 cells. *J Nutr Sci Vitaminol (Tokyo).* 45:385–390.

Ohno, N et al. 1995. Enhancement of LPS triggered TNF-alpha (tumor necrosis factor-alpha) production by 1-3 beta-D-glucan in mice. *Biol Pharm Bull.* 18:126–133.

Okazaki, M et al. 1995. Structure-activity relationship of 1-3 beta-D-glucans in the induction of cytokine production from macrophages, *in vitro. Biol Pharm Bull.* 18:1320-1327.

Yokota, M. 1992. Observatory trial of anti-obesity activity of maitake (*Grifola frondosa*). *Anshin.* 7:202–204.

Chapter Seven

Han, SB et al. 1999. The inhibitory effect of polysaccharides isolated from *Phellinus linteus* on tumor growth and metastasis. *Immunopharmacology.* 42:157–164.

Kim, HM et al. 1996. Stimulation of humoral and cell-mediated immunity by polysaccharide from mushroom *Phellinus linteus. Int J Immunopharmaco.* 18:295–303.

Ying, J et al. 1987. *Icones of Medicinal Fungi from China.* Beijing, China: Science Press.

Chapter Eight

Hayakawa, K et al. 1993. Effect of Krestin (PSK) as adjuvant treatment on the prognosis after radical radiotherapy in patients with non-small cell lung cancer. *Anticancer Res.* 13:1815–1820.

Lino, Y et al. 1995. Immunochemotherapies vs. chemotherapy as adjuvant treatment after curative resection of operable breast cancer. *Anticancer Res.* 15: 2907–2912.

Liu, J et al. 1999. Phase III clinical trial for *Yun Zhi* polysaccharopeptide (PSP) capsules. In *Advanced Research in PSP*, ed. Q. Yang. Hong Kong: Hong Kong Association for Health Care Ltd.

Nakazato, H et al. 1994. Efficacy of immunochemotherapy as adjuvant treatment after curative resection of gastric cancer. *Lancet.* 343:1122–1126.

Sun, Z et al. 1999. The ameliorative effect of PSP on the toxic and side reaction of chemo- and radiotherapy of cancers. In *Advanced Research in PSP*, ed. Q. Yang. Hong Kong: Hong Kong Association for Health Care Ltd.

Yang Q. 1999. *PSP and Its Clinical Research.* Hong Kong: Publication of the Hong Kong Association for Health Care Ltd.

Chapter Nine

Ito, M et al. 1999. Anti-tumor activity of hot-water extract of *Hericium erinaceus* (yamabushitake). *Nat Med.* 53:263–265.

Mizuno, T. 1995. Yamabushitake, *Hericium erinaceum* [*sic*]: Bioactive substances and medical utilization. *Food Rev Int.* 11:173–178.

Mizuno, T. 1999. Bioactive substances in *Hericium erinaceus* (bull.: fr) pers. (yamabushitake), and its medicinal utilization. *Int J Med Mushrooms.* 1:105–119.

Xu, HM et al. 1994. Immunomodulatory function of polysaccharide of *Hericium erinaceus* (article in Chinese). *Chung kuo chung his i chieh ho tsa chih.* 14:427–428.

Chapter Ten

Chihara, G et al. 1970. Fractionation and purification of the polysaccharides with marked anti-tumor activity, especially Lentinan from *Lentinus edodes* (Berk.) Sing., an edible mushroom. *Cancer Res.* 30:2776–2781.

Gordon, M et al. 1998. A placebo-controlled trial of the immune modulator, lentinan, in HIV-positive patients: a phase I/II trial. *J Med.* 29:305–330.

Hirasawa, M. 1999. Three kinds of antibacterial substances from *Lentinus edodes* (Berk.) Sing (shiitake, an edible mushroom). *Int J Antimicrob Agents.* 11:151–157.

Ikekawa, T et al. 1969. Anti-tumor activity of aqueous extracts of edible mushrooms. *Cancer Res.* 29:734–735.

Shouji, N. 2000. Anticaries effect of a component from shiitake (an edible mushroom). *Caries Res.* 34:94–98.

Chapter Twelve

Holliday, J et al. Clinical trial of a mixture of six medicinal mushroom extracts. *Submitted for publication.*

Kabir, Y et al. 1989. Dietary mushrooms reduce blood pressure in spontaneously hypertensive rats (SHR). *J Nutr Sci Vitaminol (Tokyo).* 35:91–94.

Raverat, Gwen. 1991. *Period Piece.* East Lansing, MI: University of Michigan Press.

Index